Beta Thalassemia

Edited by Marwa Zakaria and Tamer Hassan

Published in London, United Kingdom

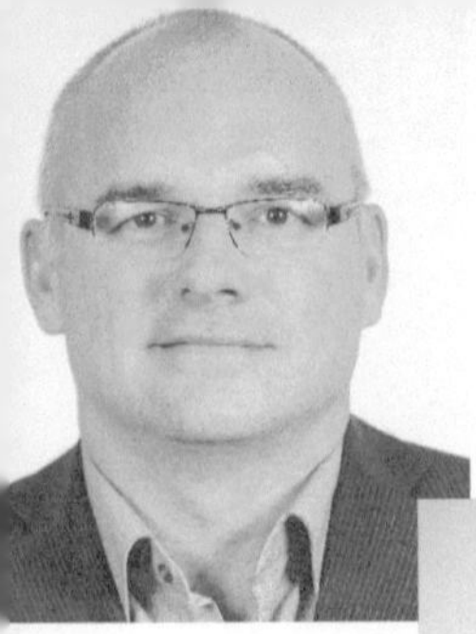
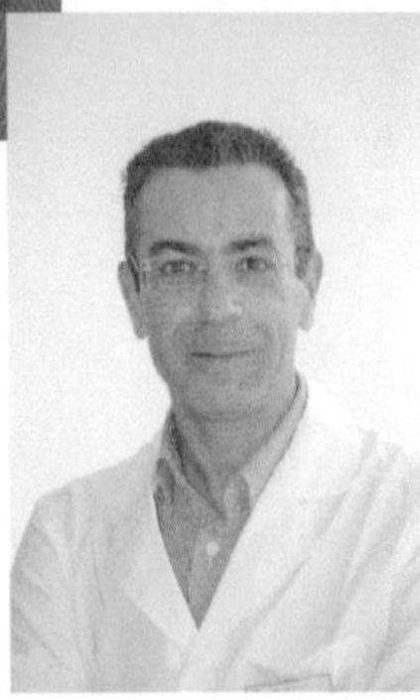
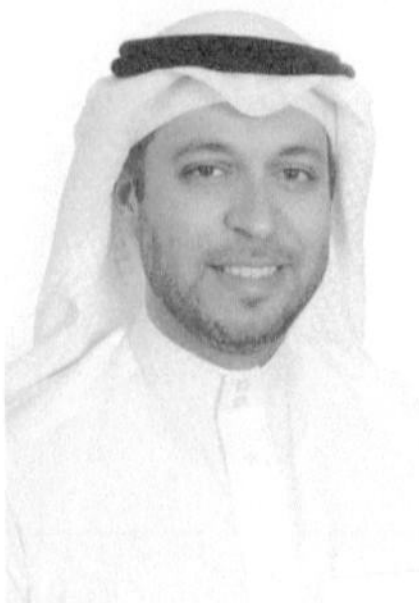
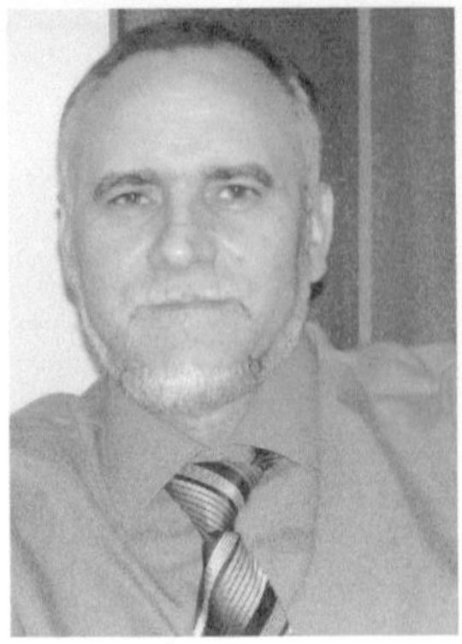
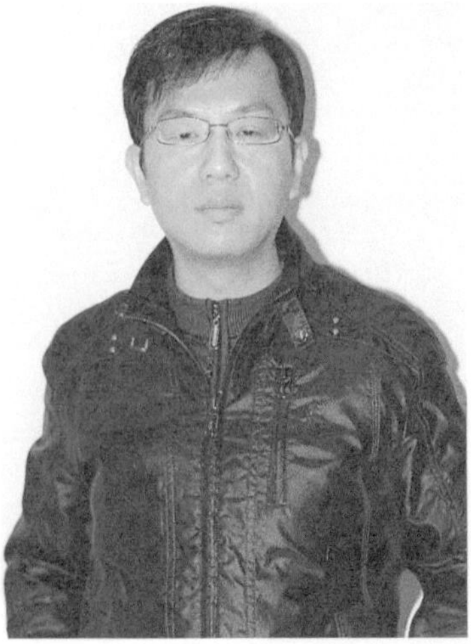
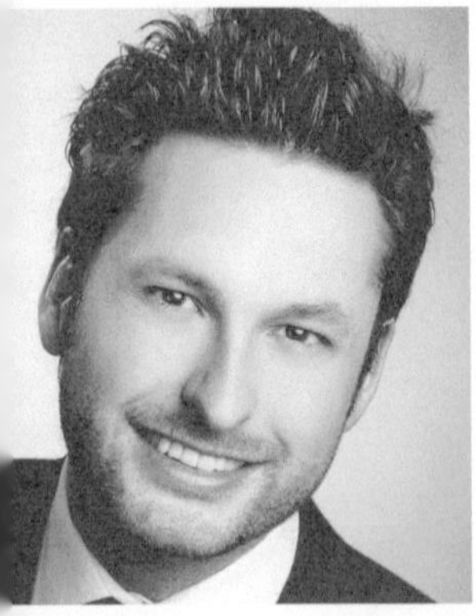
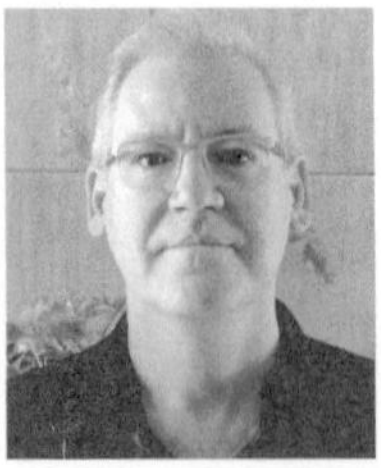

IntechOpen

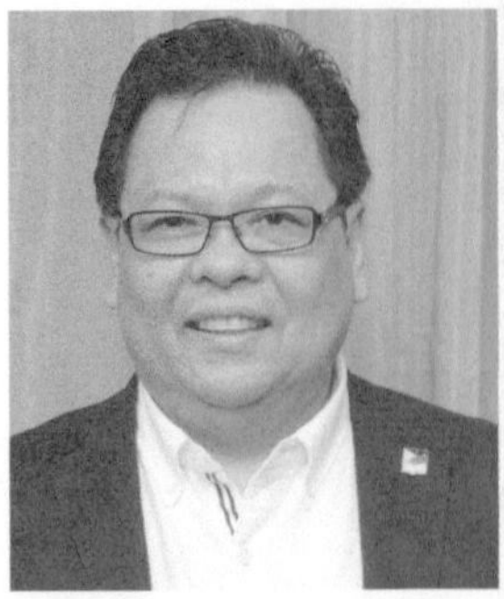
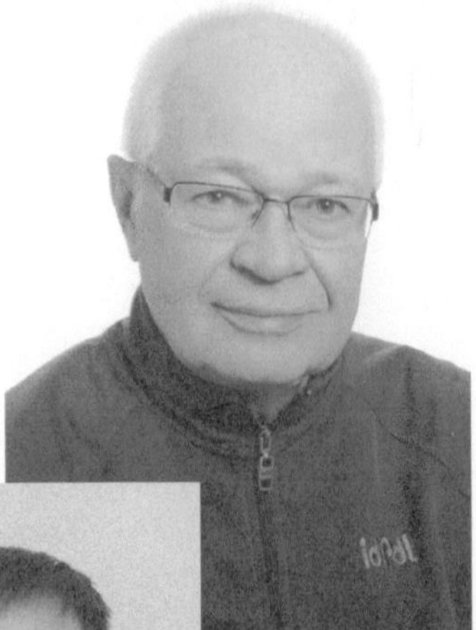
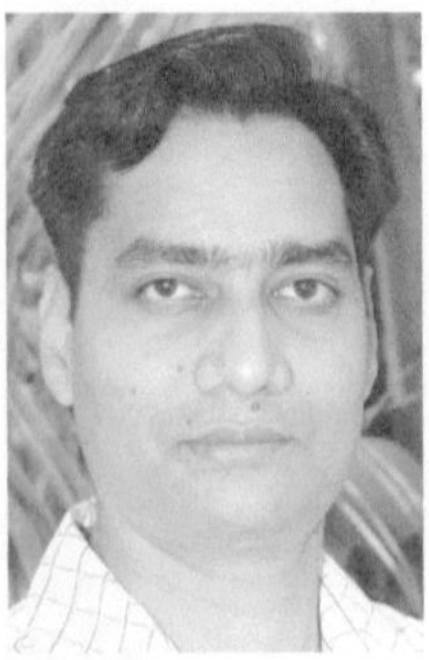
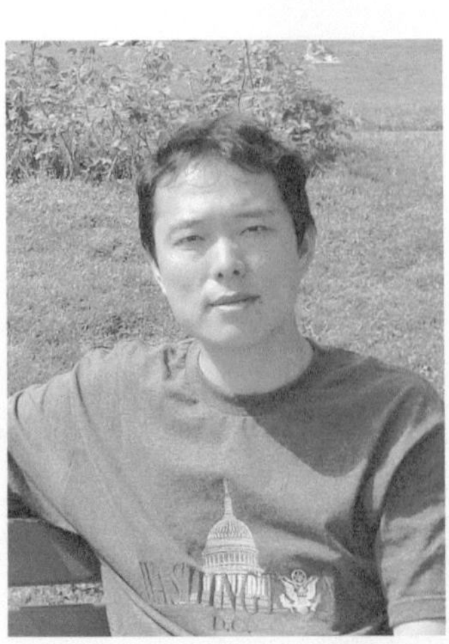
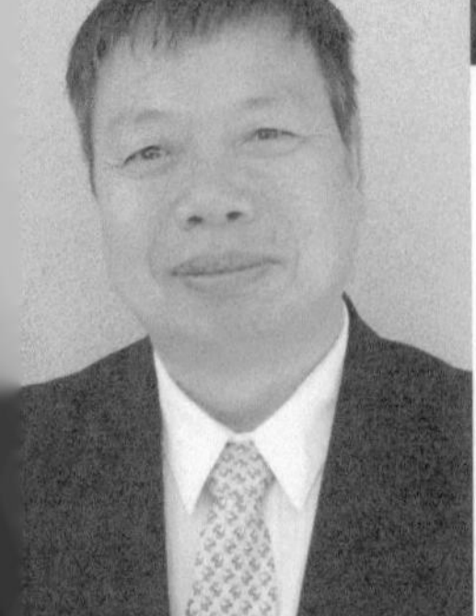
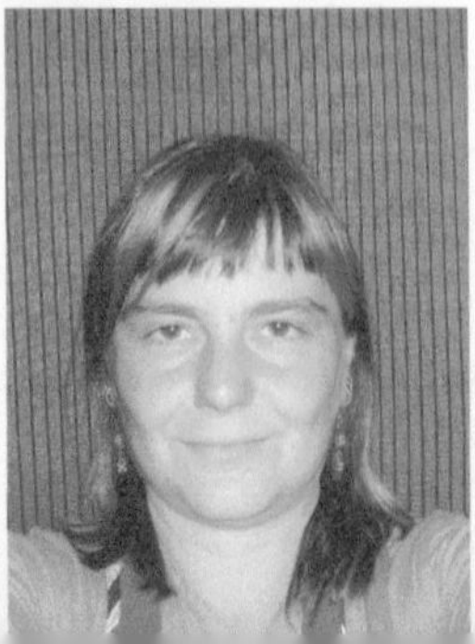

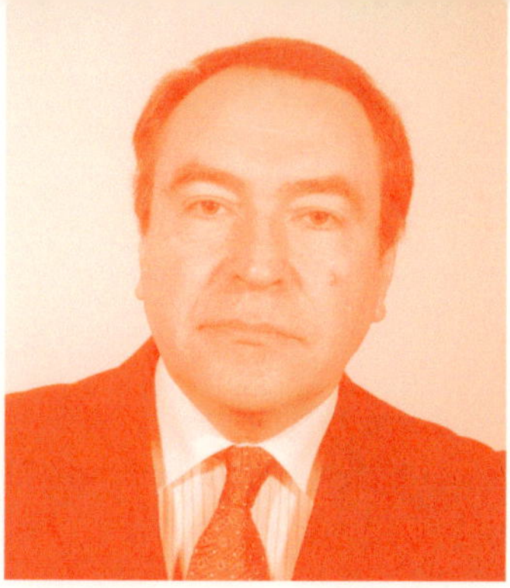
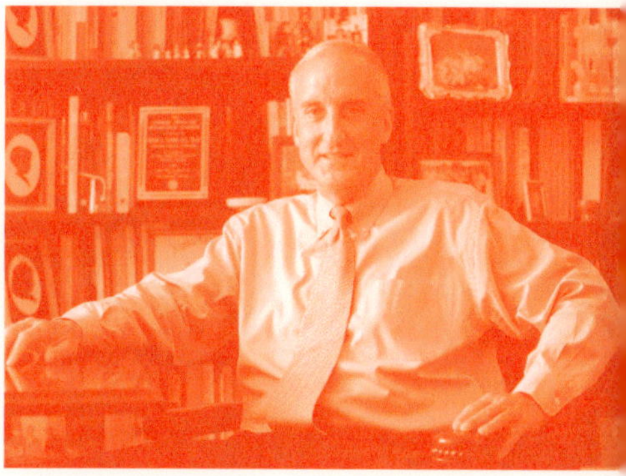
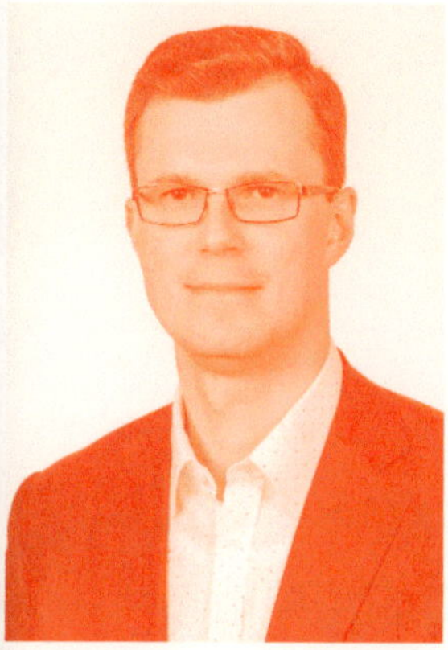
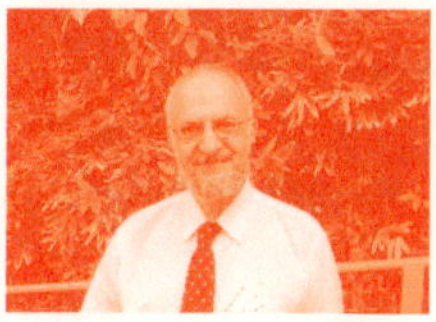
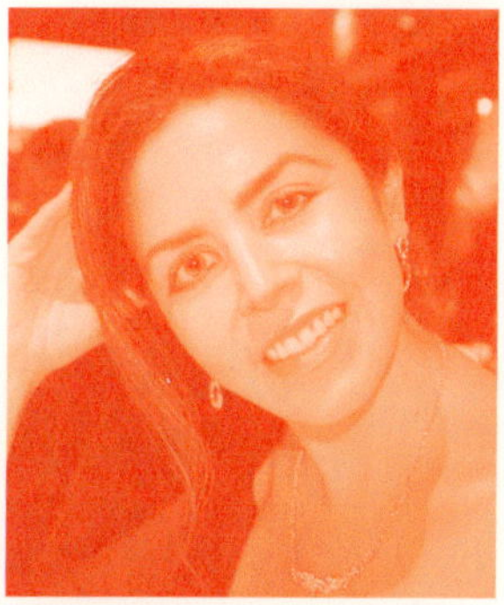

Supporting open minds since 2005

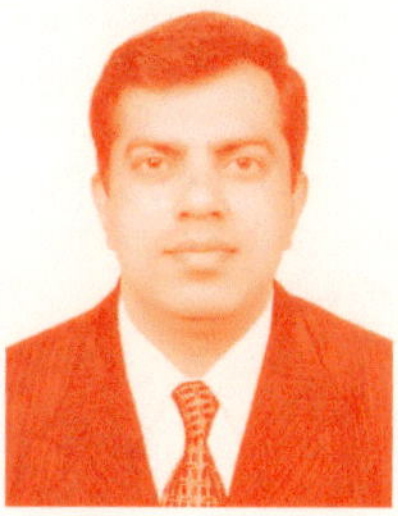
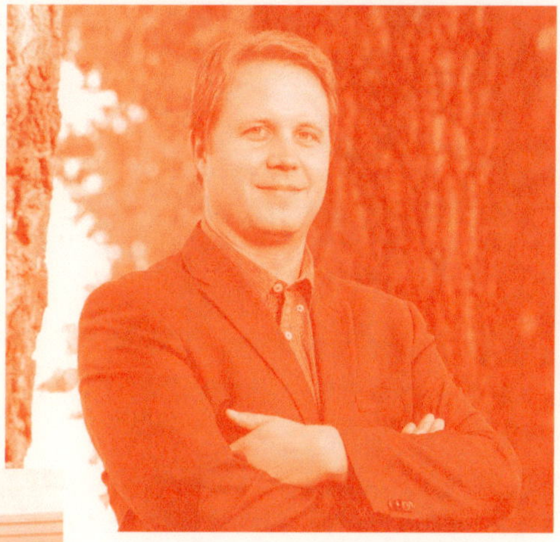
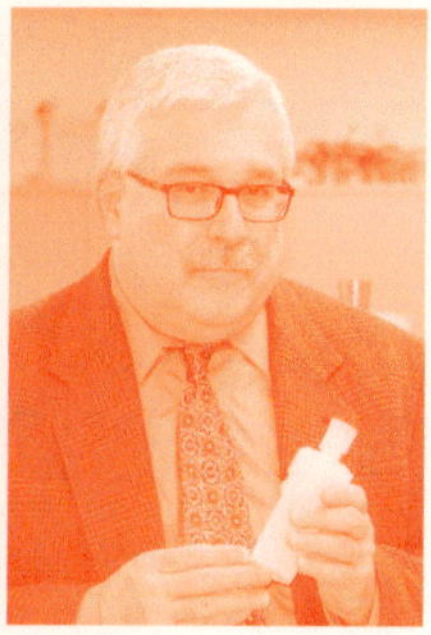
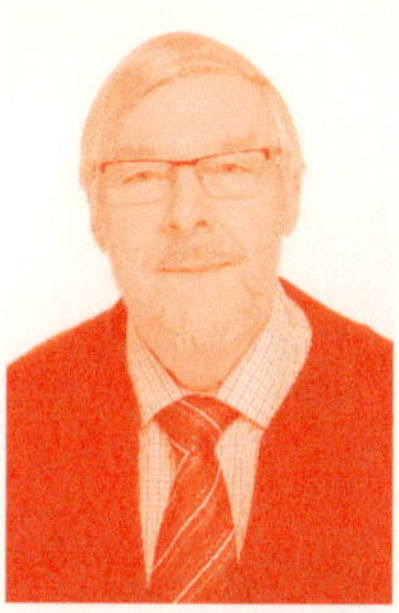
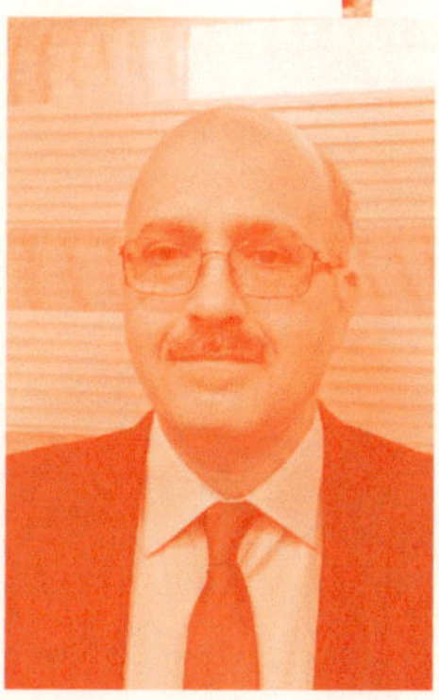
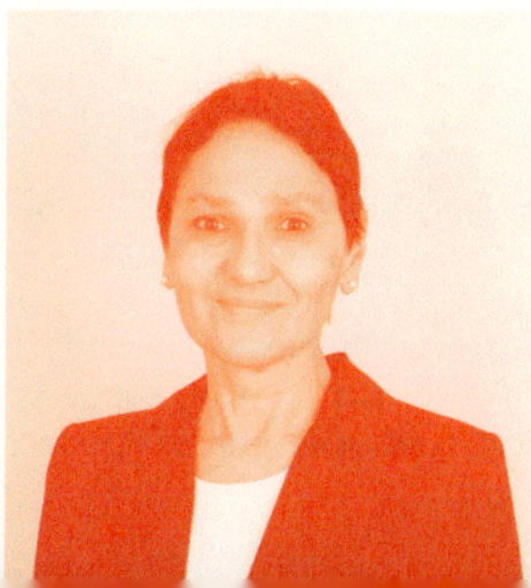
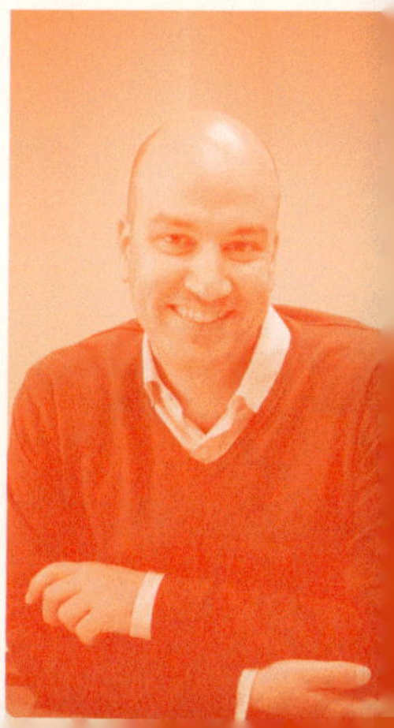

Beta Thalassemia
http://dx.doi.org/10.5772/intechopen.78823
Edited by Marwa Zakaria and Tamer Hassan

Contributors
Thanusak Tatu, Nadia Maria Sposi, Rungrote Natesirinilkul, Mark D. Scott, Somdet Srichairatanakool, Pimpisid Koonyosying, Suthat Fucharoen, Michela Grosso, Marianna De Martino, Raffaele Sessa, Maria Rosaria Storino, Mariarosaria Giuliano, Silvia Trombetti, Paola Izzo, Rosa Catapano, Alessandra Lo Bianco, Marwa Zakaria, Tamer Hasan

First published in London, United Kingdom, 2020 by IntechOpen
IntechOpen is the global imprint of INTECHOPEN LIMITED, registered in England and Wales, registration number: 11086078, 5 Princes Gate Court, London, SW7 2QJ, United Kingdom
Printed in Croatia

British Library Cataloguing-in-Publication Data
A catalogue record for this book is available from the British Library

Additional hard and PDF copies can be obtained from orders@intechopen.com

Beta Thalassemia
Edited by Marwa Zakaria and Tamer Hassan
p. cm.
Print ISBN 978-1-83880-586-9
Online ISBN 978-1-83880-587-6
eBook (PDF) ISBN 978-1-83880-588-3

For EU product safety concerns:
IN TECH d.o.o., Prolaz Marije Krucifikse Kozulić 3, 51000 Rijeka, Croatia, info@intechopen.com or visit our website at intechopen.com.

Meet the editors

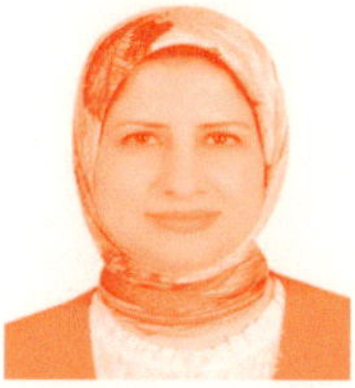

Marwa Zakaria is an active member in SIOP, EHA and HAA. His professional training and workshops include ICH GCP, EHA-master class and bite size master class. He has received training from Wilkins-Barrick Society of Neurooncology (SNO), Morocco and Training Program in Pediatric Nutrition (School of Medicine Boston University 2017). He was awarded the International Preceptorship in thalassemia (Beirut, September 2015). His international scholarships and awards include SIOP Scholarship, EHA-HOPE in 2017 and 2018 respectively. He has been the guest speaker at numerous pediatric oncology and hematology meetings and had over 20 international research publications in the field of pediatrics. He is the chief editor of two online books and author of four online book chapters. He is the reviewer for international and national peer-reviewed journals (Medicine (Baltimore), IntechOpen Publisher, Frontiers in Pediatrics, Molecular Medicine Reports, and Zagazig University Medical Journal). He is the sub-investigator in 7 international trials.

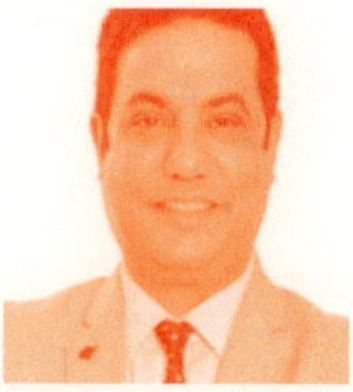

An active member at EHA, SIOP, and HAA, Tamer Hassan has had over 50 international research publications in Pediatrics. He has authored four online book chapters and been the coeditor of two online books. His professional training and workshops include ICH GCP online Training, training in 10th international educational course on thalassemia, Cyprus 2006, training in pediatric stem cell transplantation unit in Ulm University, completion of EHA master class and bite size master class 2016 and 2017 respectively. He has been awarded many international scholarships including SIOP, EHA-HOPE, Hemophilia Preceptorship in Saint Luc Hospital, Belgium, ITP Preceptorship in Dmitry Rogachev National Research Center, Moscow. He is an academic editor for the Medicine (Baltimore) Journal and a reviewer for many international journals (Hemophilia, Medicine, Oncology Letters, Child Neurology). He is the primary investigator in 3 international clinical trials and sub-investigator in 12 international trials.

Contents

Preface

This book on beta thalassemia is the first edition and has been a wonderful opportunity to bring together pediatric hematology experts from different communities. The book is designed to be a first step for better practice in the treatment of beta thalassemia. Basic and up-to-date knowledge are included in this book.

Six contributors and two editors participated in writing this book. The book is divided into four sections: Introduction to Beta Thalassemia, Updates of Beta Thalassemia, Pathophysiology of Beta Thalassemia and Diagnosis of Beta Thalassemia. Many tables and illustrations are included for quick reference in the clinical setting.

Section I focuses on the general introduction and a quick overview of beta thalassemia. Section II highlights the updates in diagnosis and treatment of beta thalassemia. Section III illustrates the pathophysiology dilemma of this disease. Section IV displays the diagnostic tools and work up of this disease.

The editors of this beta thalassemia book want to recognize, thank, and acknowledge everyone who participated in writing this book. We are profoundly aware of the personal time and commitment that was devoted to make this an outstanding resource and we are grateful. It is our hope that all healthcare, academic and clinical practitioners of advanced clinical practice will find this publication useful, and that it will enrich knowledge and improve care for children and adolescents with beta thalassemia.

Marwa Zakaria
Associate professor of Pediatrics and Pediatric Hematology and Oncology,
Pediatric Department,
Zagazig University,
Egypt

Tamer Hassan
Professor of Pediatrics and Pediatric Hematology and Oncology,
Pediatric Department,
Zagazig University,
Egypt

Section 1

Introduction to Beta Thalassemia

Chapter 1

Introductory Chapter: β-Thalassemia

Marwa Zakaria and Tamer Hassan

1. What we need to know about β-thalassemia

Thalassemia is a hereditary, autosomal recessive blood disorder due to partial or complete deficiency in the synthesis of or β-globin chains (β-thalassemia) or α-globin chains (α-thalassemia) that compose the major adult hemoglobin resulting in chronic hemolytic state.

β-Thalassemia is caused by mutations in the HBB gene resulting in decrease of the production of β chain leading to excessive accumulation of unpaired α chains that aggregate and precipitates along the red cell membranes, causing their damage and resulting in intravascular hemolysis. Also, premature destruction of erythroid precursors results in intramedullary death and ineffective erythropoiesis and a short lifespan of mature RBCs in the circulation. Frequent RBC transfusion is the main supportive therapy, leading to excessive accumulation of iron (iron overload), a condition that is exacerbated by excessive hemolysis and the increased iron reabsorption secondary to ineffective erythropoiesis.

Excessive iron is toxic and catalyzes the generation of reactive oxygen species, which in excess are toxic, causing damage to numerous body organs such as the heart and liver as well as the endocrine system. Herein, we represent an overview on thalassemia regarding the underlying pathophysiology of the disease, clinical presentations, and potential therapeutic modalities for the amelioration of its complications, as well as new modalities that may provide a cure for the disease. Thanks to the significant improvement in therapy, patients with β-thalassemia may reach an advanced age.

1.1 β-Thalassemia: types and clinical presentation

In the homozygous state of β-thalassemia which is known as thalassemia major represented with severe, transfusion-dependent anemia within the first 2 years of life. Also associated with skeletal abnormalities and poor growth, in the heterozygous state of β-thalassemia (trait or minor) causes mild to moderate microcytic anemia and not require any specific management. On the other hand, patients in whom clinical severity of the disease lies between that of thalassemia major and thalassemia trait are classified as having β-thalassemia intermedia and require only periodic blood transfusions under special circumstances [1]. Numerous different genotypes are associated with β-thalassemia intermedia, such as HbE which is a common Hb variant found in Southeast Asia, and this variant is included in the beta thalassemia category of diseases. Also, HbS (sickle cell disease) can be presented clinically with severe anemia [2].

Repeated blood transfusions resulting in excessive iron deposition and generation of ROS is a leading cause of morbidity and mortality, in those patients [3].

1.2 Removal of excess iron

Removal of blood (phlebotomy) is used to remove excess iron in patients with normal Hb levels, such as in patients with hereditary hemochromatosis, where iron overload is caused by mutations in the iron homeostasis system [4].

Most other patients with iron overload are anemic (Hb < 10 g/dL) and, therefore, particularly those who are transfusion dependent, phlebotomy would not be optimum and will require iron chelation therapy to decrease iron overload [5].

1.3 Iron chelators

Each unit of transfused red blood cells contains approximately 200 mg of elemental iron. In addition to anemia and ineffective erythropoiesis down-regulates the synthesis of hepcidin, so the use of iron chelators is mandatory to remove excess iron from the plasma as well as from tissues through binding the cheatable, labile, iron form and enhancing its excretion through the body excreta.

Three chelation agents are approved for use in the United States. Deferoxamine, the first to be used, is given by continuous intravenous infusion or slow subcutaneous, infusion through a portable pump. Its main disadvantage is poor compliance secondary to its mode of administration [6].

Deferiprone is an oral iron chelator effective in removing excess iron from the organs and mainly from the heart. The main potential complication is neutropenia that may rarely be followed by agranulocytosis. A liquid formulation has been recently introduced [7].

Deferasirox is available as oral dispersible tablets and is considered as an effective oral chelator, and it reduces liver iron concentration and serum ferritin levels. Deferasirox binds iron with high affinity in a 2:1 ratio. Its main side effects are GIT upsets in the form of abdominal pain, nausea, diarrhea, liver, and kidney dysfunction as well as skin rash. A new formulation of film-coated tablets are now available with better compliance, as it can be taken with a light meal [8].

1.3.1 Shuttle mechanism

The efficacy of chelation may be improved by the use of a combination of chelators. For example, deferiprone may mobilize iron from tissues into the circulation, where deferoxamine binds and facilitates its excretion in the urine this is what is called (the "shuttle mechanism") [9].

1.4 Dyserythropoiesis

Chronic anemia in addition to associated hypoxia in β-thalassemia stimulates excessive RBC production which is mediated through release of erythropoietin, the main erythropoietic stimulating hormone. This attempt is called "stress erythropoiesis" that passes through four steps: expansion of erythroid progenitors, accelerated erythroid differentiation, maturation arrest, and apoptosis. Many other factors, for example, transforming growth factor-β and activin receptor-II trap ligands contribute to this phenomenon. Binding of EPO to its surface receptor on erythroid precursors activates transduction pathways, including Jak2/Stat5, which inhibit apoptosis and stimulates proliferation as well as differentiation of the new cells. However, this operation is futile termed ineffective erythropoiesis due to oxidative stress-increased apoptosis and abortive differentiation [10].

Recent advances in understanding the molecular mechanism involved in two critical steps of dyserythropoiesis are paving the way to new alternative therapeutic targets.

1.5 Novel therapeutic modalities

Several therapeutic modalities aimed at reducing the dyserythropoiesis in thalassemia are currently under research. For example, activin receptor-II trap ligands, JAK2 inhibitors, induction of the Hsp70 chaperone machinery, reducing α-globin synthesis, and stimulation of HbF production [11–15].

1.5.1 Gene modification approach

The hematopoietic stem cells of the affected individual are subjected to gene editing techniques ex vivo and then reinjected again to the patient for reconstitution [16].

To increase the production of γ-globin lentiviral vectors that express a zinc finger protein has been used in order to carry microRNAs that silence its repressors or interacts with the promoter of the γ-globin gene 80 [17].

Genome editing of the promoter of BCL11A can be accomplished by several nucleases, such as engineered zinc finger nucleases (ZFNs), transcription activator-like effector nucleases (TALENs), and clustered regularly interspaced short palindromic repeats linked to Cas9 nucleases (CRISPR-Cas9) (**Figure 1**) [18]. Recently, it has been shown that ZFN-driven BCL11A enhancer ablation leads to increased production of HbF in erythroid progenitors derived hematopoietic stem cell from β-thalassemia patient which could be used for autologous transplantation [19]. Similarly, CRISPR-Cas9-mediated BCL11A enhancer inactivation in a human adult-stage erythroid cell line can achieve the same results [20].

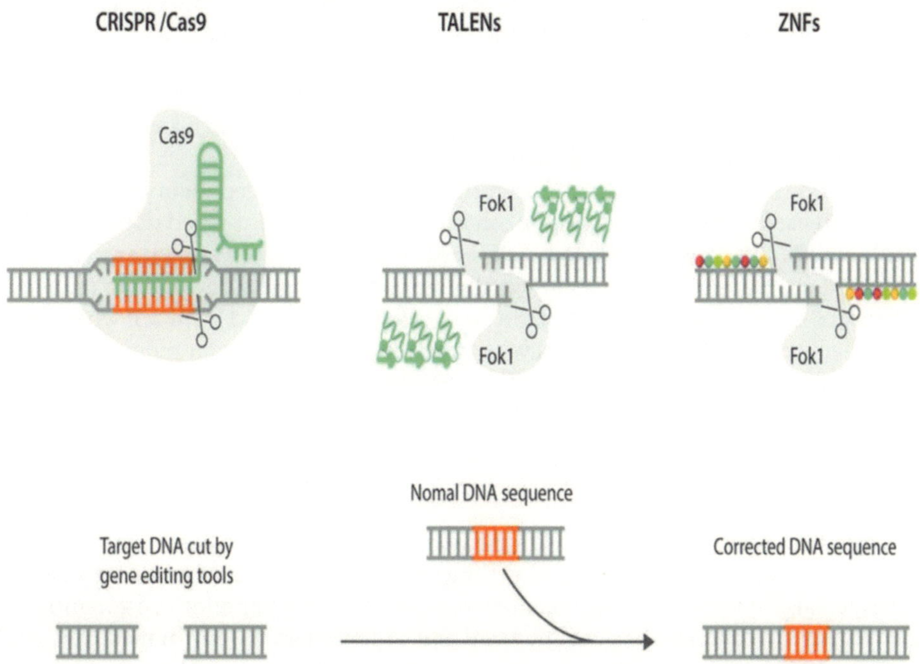

Figure 1.
Mechanism of gene editing.

1.5.2 Gene therapy

Currently, gene therapy represents a novel therapeutic promise, after many years of extensive preclinical research for the optimization of gene transfer regimen. This is mediated through autologous transplantation of genetically modified hematopoietic stem cells, clinical trials being held worldwide have revealed that, by re-establishing effective hemoglobin production, patients may be rendered transfusion- and chelation-independent and escapes the immunological sequel that normally accompany allogeneic hematopoietic stem cell transplantation.

The approach of gene therapy has focused on two mechanisms: first, increasing the production of β-globin by the addition of a normal gene or correction of the mutated gene; and second, increasing the production of γ-globin by the addition of its gene, overexpression of its endogenous activating transcription factors, and silencing of its repressors. Studies of gene therapy have utilized mainly lentivirus vectors in experimental systems, including cultured CD34 HSCs from β-thalassemia patients and β-thalassemia mouse models. Yet the safety profile of such technologies is still uncertain [16].

Genomic editing has been demonstrated to modify the β-globin gene. Thus, TALEN-mediated gene correction has been used in induced HSCs from β-thalassemia patients [21].

1.5.3 Allogeneic hematopoietic stem cell transplantation

Currently, allogeneic stem cell transplant [allo-SCT] remains the only curative option for the majority of patients with β-thalassemia major before development of iron overload complications [22].

Patients with β-thalassemia major who have good risk features are reasonable to anticipate a greater than 90% chance of successful transplant outcome, even patients with high risk features, success rates are approaching 80%.

Challenging in allo-HSCT in high-risk patients is mainly related to graft rejection and risk of transplant-related mortality but nowadays novel modified or reduced-intensity conditioning regimens are used to improve the transplantation outcome in β-thalassemia patients with cheerful results [23].

Traditionally, completely matched human leukocyte antigen identical siblings have been used as donors, and on the other hand, matched unrelated donors have also been tried in patients with low risk. Bone marrow has been known as the preferred choice of stem cells in non-malignant hematological disorders to reduce the risk of GVHD but peripheral blood stem cell graft and cord stem cell when used have been reported to be associated with faster engraftment, lower requirement of blood product support in the peri-transplant period, and a low incidence of graft rejection in patients with low-risk [24, 25].

1.6 Preventive strategies for thalassemia

Despite the great advances in management tools used in β-thalassemia to improve the cure rate of the disease, yet the incidence rate of the disease is increasing especially in underdeveloped countries where the prevalence of consanguineous marriage is high and low level of standard and sometimes shortage in medical resources and supply that limit the early detection of carrier state. Therefore, the prevention of the homozygous state presents a big challenging issue. Prevention including prenatal diagnosis, carrier detections, molecular diagnosis, and genetic counseling is strongly needed.

1.6.1 Prenatal diagnosis

Recently, prenatal diagnosis is carried out for couples at risk, either in first trimester through obtaining fetal material by chorionic villus sampling or in the second trimester through cordocentesis or amniocentesis.

One of the main successful procedures in prenatal diagnosis is to study the fetal erythroid cells and detection of globin gene mutations. As the first primitive erythroblasts appear in embryonic bloodstream around the 4–5 weeks gestations, so obtaining fetal material by aspiration of coelomic fluid (celocentesis) followed by selection of embryo-fetal erythroid precursors by an anti-CD71 microbeads method or by direct micromanipulator pickup of the cells has been extensively improved and used by several groups [26, 27].

Nowadays, the possibility of cheaper and safer prenatal diagnosis facilities has emerged. Fetal-derived genetic material (cells or cell free DNA) can be obtained from the maternal blood and analyzed, which is considered a non-invasive maneuver with no risk of miscarriage and needs neither complicated procedures nor highly trained personnel for sampling. This allows future screening for thalassemia as well as other genetic diseases [28].

Detection or exclusion of inherited fetal mutations is one of the most important approaches that focuses on detection of mutation that are absent from mother's

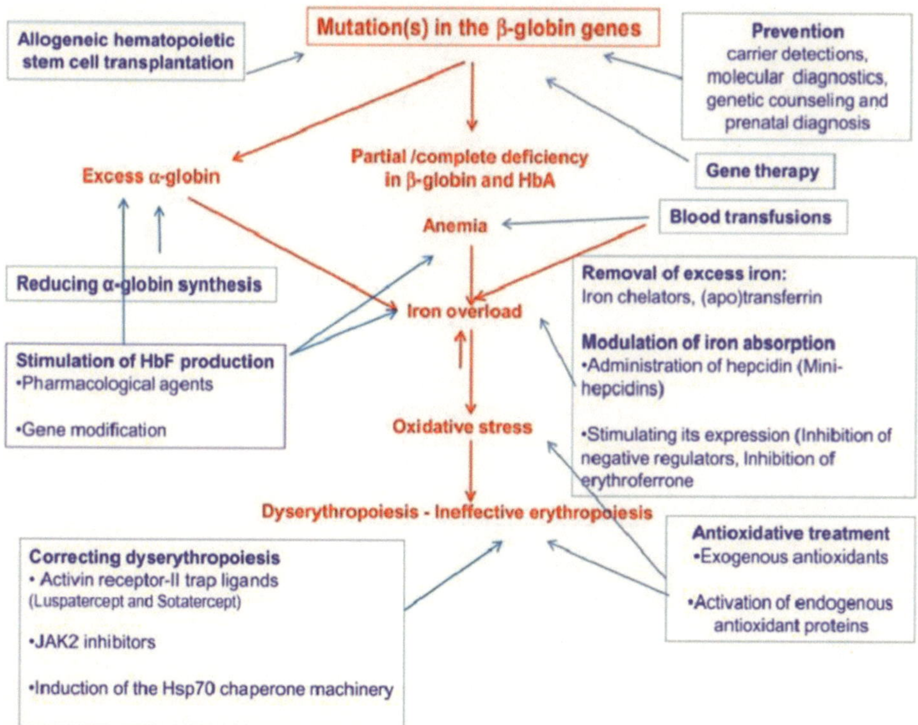

Figure 2.
Beta-thalassemia: causes, symptoms, and therapeutic modalities. Causes and symptoms are marked in red; and therapeutic modalities are marked in blue.

genome that requires DNA quantifications with high sensitivity. Even when the parents have the identical mutation, the relative mutation/haplotype approach might detect this fetal mutation [29].

1.6.2 Pre-implantation genetic diagnosis

One of the promising approaches is pre-implantation genetic diagnosis of cells (PGD) usually single cells, which had been biopsied from oocytes/zygotes or embryos obtained by in vitro fertilization and testing it for specific genetic abnormality. PGD assists couples to avoid birth of an affected child and limit the needs for abortion. This maneuver aims at delivery of an unaffected newborn. PGD helps to identify unaffected embryos for transfer to the uterus [30].

Lastly to conclude, the most likely approach to reduce the patients' load is efficient prevention, carrier detection, prenatal diagnosis, and genetic counseling, and here, we summarize causes, symptoms, and therapeutic modalities in β-thalassemia as illustrated in **Figure 2**.

Author details

Marwa Zakaria* and Tamer Hassan
Faculty of Medicine, Zagazig University, Zagazig, Egypt

*Address all correspondence to: marwazakaria12@yahoo.com

References

[1] Rund D, Rachmilewitz E. Beta-thalassemia. The New England Journal of Medicine. 2005;**353**:1135-1146. DOI: 10.1056/NEJMra050436

[2] Kan YW, Nathan DG. Mild thalassemia: The result of interactions of alpha and beta thalassemia genes. The Journal of Clinical Investigation. 1970;**49**:635-642. DOI: 10.1172/JCI106274

[3] Porter JB, Garbowski M. The pathophysiology of transfusional iron overload. Hematology/Oncology Clinics of North America. 2014;**28**:683-701. DOI: 10.1016/j.hoc.2014.04.003

[4] Rombout-Sestrienkova E, van Kraaij MG, Koek GH. How we manage patients with hereditary haemochromatosis. British Journal of Haematology. 2016;**175**:759-770. DOI: 10.1111/bjh.14376

[5] Leitch HA, Fibach E, Rachmilewitz E. Toxicity of iron overload and iron overload reduction in the setting of hematopoietic stem cell transplantation for hematologic malignancies. Critical Reviews in Oncology/Hematology. 2017;**113**:156-170. DOI: 10.1016/j.critrevonc.2017.03.002

[6] Haghpanah S, Zarei T, Zahedi Z, et al. Compliance and satisfaction with Deferasirox (Exjade®) compared with deferoxamine in patients with transfusion-dependent beta-thalassemia. Hematology. 2014;**19**:187-191. DOI: 10.1179/1607845413Y.0000000121

[7] Chuansumrit A, Songdej D, Sirachainan N, et al. Safety profile of a liquid formulation of deferiprone in young children with transfusion-induced iron overload: A 1-year experience. Paediatrics and International Child Health. 2016;**36**:209-213. DOI: 10.1179/2046905515Y.0000000040

[8] Taher AT, Origa R, Perrotta S, et al. New film-coated tablet formulation of Deferasirox is well tolerated in patients with thalassemia or lower-risk MDS: Results of the randomized, phase II ECLIPSE study. American Journal of Hematology. 2017;**92**:420-428. DOI: 10.1002/ajh.24668

[9] Vlachodimitropoulou Koumoutsea E, Garbowski M, Porter J. Synergistic intracellular iron chelation combinations: Mechanisms and conditions for optimizing iron mobilization. British Journal of Haematology. 2015;**170**:874-883. DOI: 10.1111/bjh.13512

[10] Dussiot M, Maciel TT, Fricot A, et al. An activin receptor IIA ligand trap corrects ineffective erythropoiesis in β-thalassemia. Nature Medicine. 2014;**20**:398-407. DOI: 10.1038/nm.3468

[11] Motta I, Scaramellini N, Cappellini MD. Investigational drugs in phase I and phase II clinical trials for thalassemia. Expert Opinion on Investigational Drugs. 2017;**26**:793-802. DOI: 10.1080/13543784.2017.1335709

[12] Casu C, Oikonomidou PR, Lo Presti V, et al. Potential therapeutic applications of JAK2 inhibitors and HIF2a-ASO for the treatment of beta-thalassemia intermedia and major. American Journal of Hematology. 2017;**92**:E221-E221. DOI: 10.3324/haematol.2017.181511

[13] Guillem F, Dussiot M, Causse S, et al. XPO1 (exportin-1) is a major regulator of human erythroid differentiation. Potential clinical applications to decrease ineffective erythropoiesis of beta-thalassemia. Blood. 2015;**126**:2368. DOI: 10.1155/2013/394295

[14] Mettananda S, Fisher CA, Sloane-Stanley JA, et al. Selective silencing of α-globin by the histone demethylase inhibitor IOX1: A potentially new pathway for treatment of β-thalassemia. Haematologica. 2017;**102**:e80-e84. DOI: 10.3324/haematol.2016

[15] Sripichai O, Fucharoen S. Fetal hemoglobin regulation in β-thalassemia: Heterogeneity, modifiers and therapeutic approaches. Expert Review of Hematology. 2016;**9**:1129-1137. DOI: 10.1080/17474086.2016.1255142

[16] Smith EC, Orkin SH. Hemoglobin genetics: Recent contributions of GWAS and gene editing. Human Molecular Genetics. 2016;**25**:R99-R105. DOI: 10.1093/hmg/ddw170

[17] Guda S, Brendel C, Renella R, et al. miRNA-embedded shRNAs for lineage-specific BCL11A knockdown and hemoglobin F induction. Molecular Therapy. 2015;**23**:1465-1474. DOI: 10.1038/mt.2015.113

[18] McNutt M. Breakthrough to genome editing. Science. 2015;**350**:1445. DOI: 10.1126/science.aae0479

[19] Reik A, Chang K, Vierstra J, et al. 53. From GWAS to the clinic: Genome editing the human BCL11A erythroid enhancer for fetal globin elevation in the hemoglobinopathies. Molecular Therapy. 2015;**23**:S23-S24. DOI: 10.1016/S1525-0016(16)33658-9

[20] Bauer DE, Canver MC, Smith EC, et al. Crispr-Cas9 saturating mutagenesis reveals an Achilles heel in the BCL11A erythroid enhancer for fetal hemoglobin induction (by genome editing). Blood. 2015;**126**:638. DOI: 10.1182/blood.V126.23.638.638

[21] Ma N, Liao B, Zhang H, et al. Transcription activator-like effector nuclease (TALEN)-mediated gene correction in integration-free β-thalassemia induced pluripotent stem cells. The Journal of Biological Chemistry. 2013;**288**:34671-34679. DOI: 10.1074/jbc.M113.496174

[22] Lucarelli G, Isgrò A, Sodani P, et al. Hematopoietic stem cell transplantation in thalassemia and sickle cell anemia. Cold Spring Harbor Perspectives in Medicine. 2012;**2**:a011825. DOI: 10.1101/cshperspect.a011825

[23] Gaziev J, De Angelis G, Isgro A, et al. Transplant outcomes in high-risk (class 3) patients with thalassemia treated with a modified protocol are equivalent to low/intermediate-risk (class 1/class 2) patients. Blood. 2015;**126**:620. DOI: 10.1182/blood.V126.23.620.62

[24] Angelucci E, Matthes-Martin S, Baronciani D, et al. Hematopoietic stem cell transplantation in thalassemia major and sickle cell disease: Indications and management recommendations from an international expert panel. Haematologica. 2014;**99**:811-820. DOI: 10.3324/haematol.2013.099747

[25] King AA, Kamani N, Bunin N, et al. Successful matched sibling donor marrow transplantation following reduced intensity conditioning in children with hemoglobinopathies. American Journal of Hematology. 2015;**90**:1093-1098. DOI: 10.1002/ajh.24183

[26] Giambona A, Leto F, Damiani G, et al. Identification of embryo-fetal cells in celomic fluid using morphological and short-tandem repeats analysis. Prenatal Diagnosis. 2016;**36**:973-978. DOI: 10.1002/pd.4922

[27] Avent ND, Plummer ZE, Madgett TE, et al. Post-genomics studies and their application to non-invasive prenatal diagnosis. Seminars in Fetal & Neonatal Medicine. 2008;**13**:91-98. DOI: 10.1016/j.siny.2007.12.011

[28] Li DZ, Yang YD. Invasive prenatal diagnosis of fetal thalassemia. Best Practice & Research. Clinical Obstetrics & Gynaecology. 2017;**39**:41-52. DOI: 10.1016/j.bpobgyn.2016.10.011

[29] Hudecova I, Chiu RW. Non-invasive prenatal diagnosis of thalassemias using maternal plasma cell free DNA. Best Practice & Research. Clinical Obstetrics & Gynaecology. 2017;**39**:63-73. DOI: 10.1016/j.bpobgyn.2016.10.016

[30] Traeger-Synodinos J. Pre-implantation genetic diagnosis. Best Practice & Research. Clinical Obstetrics & Gynaecology. 2017;**39**:74-88. DOI: 10.1016/j.bpobgyn.2016.10.010

Section 2

Updates in Beta Thalassemia

Chapter 2

Updates in Thalassemia

Tamer Hassan and Marwa Zakaria

Abstract

Beta-thalassemia is a genetic disease caused by mutations in the β-globin gene, resulting in partial or complete deficiency of β-chain. Deficiency of β-chain was accompanied by excess unmatched α-globin chains with subsequent dyserythropoiesis, oxidative stress, and chronic anemia. The main therapeutic option is blood transfusion that improves the anemic status but unfortunately exacerbates iron overload status. Till now, the only curative measure is allo-hematopoietic stem cell transplantation. New diagnostic and therapeutic modalities are now available. These include the preimplantation genetic diagnosis and new tools in the assessment of iron overload. Also, new therapeutic options aimed at different targets are being developed; for example, therapies that stimulate the synthesis of γ-globin and reduce the synthesis of α-globin, as well as the iron excess, dyserythropoiesis, and oxidative stress. However, the most likely ideal approach is efficient prevention, through genetic counseling, carrier detection, and prenatal diagnosis.

Keywords: β-thalassemia, genetic diagnosis, gene therapy, gene editing, new iron chelators, HSCT

1. Introduction

1.1 Updates in diagnosis

1.1.1 Preimplantation genetic diagnosis

Prenatal diagnosis (PND) services are the best practices to control prevalence of disease. Wide spread practicing of PND proved effective in reducing the number of new cases but on the other hand high abortion rate is hided, which ethically unaccepted and for many couples is not a suitable choice. Preimplantation genetic diagnosis is considered in a similar fashion to prenatal diagnosis (PGD) and is a strong alternative to conventional PND. PGD means genetic profiling of embryos prior to implantation (embryo profiling). Its main advantage is that it avoids selective pregnancy termination as the method makes it highly likely that the baby will be free of the disease under consideration. At present PGD is the only abortion free fetal diagnostic process [1].

The most important indications of PGD [1] are:

- monogenic disorders, e.g., Thalassemias;
- HLA matching (savior baby);
- cancer predisposition; and
- sex discernment.

Technical aspects (Figure 1) [2]:

1. obtaining embryos (assisted reproductive technology)
    - controlled ovarian stimulation (COH) to obtain large number of oocytes and
    - ICSI/IVF;
2. obtaining biopsy (blastomere or blastocyst biopsy);
3. genetic analysis techniques (PCR, FISH); and
4. embryo transfer and cryopreservation of surplus embryos.

Mutation testing:

PGD method to diagnose beta thalassemia was initially reported in 1998 and used either denaturing gradient gel electrophoresis or restriction enzyme digestion methods to perform the mutation analysis. The possibility of misdiagnosis due to allele drop out (ADO) and DNA contamination is considered to be the major problems associated with preimplantation genetic diagnosis [3]. Recently, the European Society of Human Reproduction and Technology (ESHRE) recommends doing both direct and indirect mutation testing using short tandem repeat (STR) linkage analysis to achieve the highest accuracy rate [4].

1.1.2 Assessment of iron overload in thalassemia

a. Well established methods for assessment of iron overload in thalassemia [5]:

- serum ferritin;
- liver biopsy for liver iron content (LIC);
- echocardiography, MUGA for cardiac iron; and
- MRI T2* for LIC and cardiac iron.

b. New methods—monitoring of liver iron overload by SQUID:

- Superconducting QUantum Interference Device (SQUID) has been recently introduced as an integral part of thalassemia care in few centers worldwide. The SQUID allows the thalassemia team to monitor iron concentration in the livers of patients and gives them a reliable tool to help adjust medication in order to avoid serious complications [6].

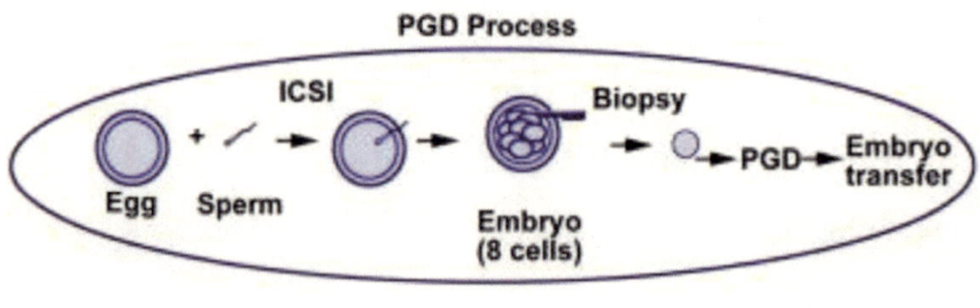

Figure 1.
Technical steps of PGD [2].

Mechanism of action of SQUID:

SQUID has high-power magnetic field. Iron interferes with the field and changes in the field are detected [6].

Advantages and disadvantages of SQUID:

Advantages and disadvantages of SQUID are listed in **Table 1** [6].

Advantages	Disadvantages
Linear correlation with LIC assessed by liver biopsy	Indirect measure of LIC
May be repeated frequently	Limited availability
	High cost
	Highly specialized: needs dedicated technician
	May underestimate LIC levels

Table 1.
Advantages and disadvantages of SQUID.

1.2 Updates in treatment

1.2.1 Gene therapy

The first obstacle against gene therapy was the extremely complex regulation of the globin genes. The second and equally important obstacle has been the lack of an optimal vector for gene transfer into quiescent hematopoietic stem cells (HSC) [7].

The first successful gene therapy for β-thalassemia major was in 2007. The process is as follow: autologous HSCs are harvested from the patient and then genetically modified with a lentiviral vector expressing a normal globin gene. After the patient has undergone appropriate conditioning therapy to destroy existing defective HSCs, the modified HSCTs are reintroduced to the patient [8].

Two large clinical trials have been recently conducted. The first one was entitled "ß-Thalassemia Major with Autologous CD34+ Hematopoietic Progenitor Cells Transduced with TNS9.3.55 a Lentiviral Vector Encoding the Normal Human ß-Globin Gene." This trial was sponsored by Memorial Sloan Kettering Cancer Center. The second one was entitled "A Study Evaluating the Efficacy and Safety of the LentiGlobin® BB305 Drug Product in Subjects with Transfusion-Dependent β-Thalassemia, who do Not Have a β0/β0 Genotype." It was sponsored by bluebird bio. Expected success awaits these clinical trials (**Figure 2**) [9].

1.2.2 Gene editing

A newer approach employs genome editing techniques, such as transcription activator-like effectors nucleases (TALEN), zinc finger nucleases (ZFN), or the clustered regularly interspaced short palindromic repeats (CRISPR) with Cas9 nuclease system. They replace the target single-mutation sites with the correct sequence, restoring the functional gene configuration. Producing a sufficiently large number of corrected genes is the major challenge with this new approach (**Figure 3**) [7].

1.2.3 Targeting ineffective erythropoiesis

A large number of preclinical and early clinical studies investigating erythropoiesis modulators are currently studied. These modulators include

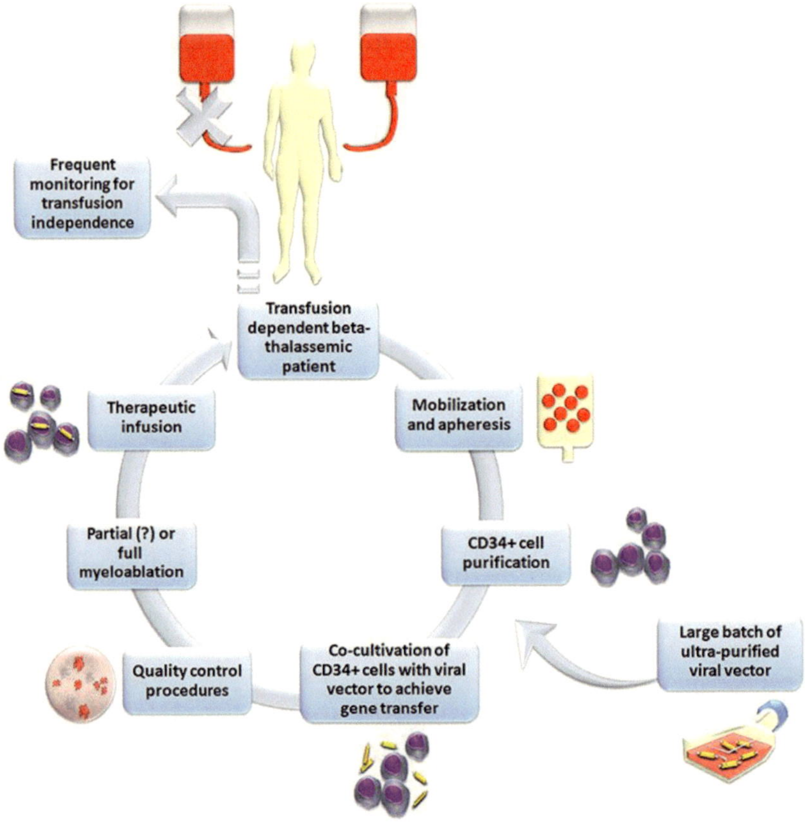

Figure 2.
Gene therapy of beta thalassemia [9].

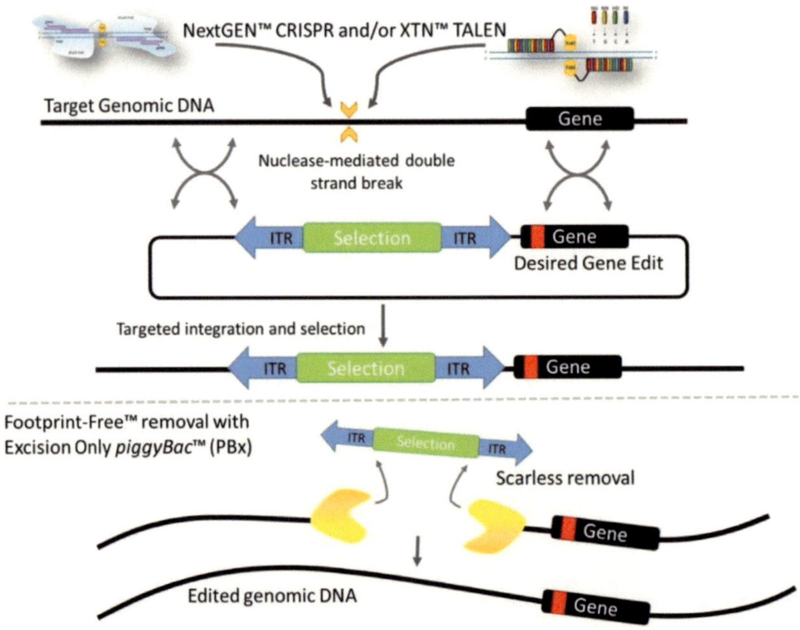

Figure 3.
Gene editing of beta thalassemia [7].

TGF-β-like molecules or inhibitors of JAK2, Foxo3 activators, HRI-Eif2ap stimulators, Prx-2 activators, HO-1 inhibitors, Hsp-70 chaperone induction and pyruvate kinase activation. These modulators could soon revolutionize the treatment of β-thalassemia and related disorders [10].

Activins, members of TGF-β family signaling, are crucial regulators of hematopoiesis and modulate various cellular responses such as differentiation, proliferation, migration, and apoptosis. They were observed to ameliorate hematologic parameters and improve hematopoiesis in preclinical and early clinical studies [11].

JAK2 plays an important role in the progression and worsening of ineffective erythropoiesis. Drugs inhibiting JAK2 activity could reverse ineffective erythropoiesis and splenomegaly [12].

1.2.4 Manipulating iron metabolism

Hepcidin is the central regulator of iron homeostasis. Hepcidin inhibitors, e.g., ERFE inhibitors are now extensively studied as a possible future treatment of iron overload. Induction of iron restriction by means of transferrin infusions, minihepcidins, or manipulation of the hepcidin pathway prevents iron overload, redistributes iron from parenchymal cells to macrophage stores, and partially controls anemia in β-thalassemic mice [13].

1.2.5 New formulation of iron chelators

Patients with transfusional iron overload usually require iron chelation therapy (ICT) to help decrease the iron burden and to prevent and/or delay long-term complications associated with iron deposition in tissues [14]. There are currently three available iron chelators.

1.2.5.1 Deferoxamine

DFO is a hexadentate iron chelator that binds iron in 1:1 complexes. It is given subcutaneously using a pump or intravenously as it is not absorbed orally. The dose ranges from 20 to 50 mg/kg/day. Though it is an effective drug, limited compliance was reported due to the inconvenience of parenteral administration as well as infectious complications [14].

1.2.5.2 Deferiprone

DFP was the first oral iron chelator to be used for transfusional iron overload. DFP is a bidentate iron chelator that forms 3:1 complexes. The dose ranges from 75 to 100 mg/kg/day divided over three doses. Treatment with DFP was associated with lower myocardial iron deposition compared to deferoxamine. The most common adverse effects of DFP include GIT disturbances, elevated liver enzymes and arthropathy. The most serious adverse event was neutropenia that was recovered after temporary discontinuation of treatment [14].

1.2.5.3 Deferasirox

DFX is another iron chelator. It is a tridentate that forms 2:1 complexes. The dose ranges from 20 to 40 mg/kg/day. DFX is a long acting iron chelator. It is given once daily which is convenient to most patients. It lacks the DFP's potentially life-threatening adverse effect of agranulocytosis. Patient Compliance and adherence to long-term chelation therapy in patients with transfusion-dependent β-thalassemia is challenging and critical to prevent iron overload-related complications. Thanks to oral iron chelators formulations that allow better compliance and improve patients and parents' adherence to the drugs. Once-daily deferasirox dispersible tablets (DT) have proven long-term efficacy and safety in patients ≥2 years old with chronic transfusional iron overload. However, barriers to optimal adherence remain, including palatability, preparation time, and requirements for fasting state. A new film-coated tablet (FCT) formulation was developed, swallowed once daily (whole/crushed) with/without a light meal [15]. Key differences between deferasirox dispersible and film coated tablets are listed in **Table 2**.

1.2.5.4 Combined iron chelators

Combined DFO and DFP chelation therapy was introduced to manage iron overload in patients with suboptimal chelation with maximum DFP doses. A shuttle mechanism was proposed to explain the synergistic effect of DFP and DFO. DFP enters cells due to its low molecular weight and removes iron, and then passes it on to DFO to be excreted in urine and stool. Other combinations like DFX & DFO and DFX & DFP were used to maximize efficacy, improve compliance and minimize the side effects [14].

1.2.6 Fetal hemoglobin induction

The main pathophysiological determinant of the severity of β-thalassemia syndromes is the extent of α/non-α globin chain imbalance. Thus in β-thalassemia, pharmacologically induced increase in γ-globin chains would be expected to decrease globin chain imbalance with consequent amelioration of clinical manifestation. Increased production of the fetal γ-globin can bind the excess α-chains to produce fetal hemoglobin and hence improve α/β-globin chain imbalance leading to more effective erythropoiesis. This partly explains the more favorable phenotype in some patients with β-thalassemia intermedia and hemoglobin E/β-thalassemia compared with transfusion-dependent β-thalassemia major [16].

Several pharmacologic compounds including: 5-azacytidine, decitabine, hydroxyurea (HU), butyrate (short-chain fatty acids), erythropoietin and short chain fatty acid derivatives (SCFAD) as fetal hemoglobin-inducing agents had encouraging results in clinical trials [16].

1.2.7 Haploidentical hematopoietic stem cell transplantation

Haploidentical transplant approach have a crucial clinical significance in patients with beta thalassemia major as it provides a graft source to almost all patients who do not have an HLA-matched donors. Haploidentical HSCT is always available and parents of children are highly motivated. Haploidentical means 50% identity and the problem is the subsequent high risk of graft versus host disease (GVHD) caused by donor T cells. Successful haploidentical HSCT depends on effective removal of donor T cells [17].

Methods of T-Cell depletion [17]:

1. CD34+ positive selection with immunomagnetic separation which leads to enrichment of stem cells;

2. CD3 depletion with immunomagnetic separation which leads to specific reduction of T cells; and

3. Addition of Alemtuzumab (anti-CD52 antibody) to the transplant bag.

	Dispersible tablet [EXJADE]	Film-coated tablet [JADENU]

Dosage forms and strengths	• White round tablet
	  ○ 125 mg
	  ○ 250 mg
	  ○ 500 mg
		• Film-coated blue oval tablet
		  ○ 90 mg (light blue)
		  ○ 180 mg (medium blue)
		  ○ 360 mg (dark blue)

Administration	• Once daily on an empty stomach ≥30 minutes before a meal
	• Stir to disperse in water, orange juice or apple juice
	  ○ 3.5 oz. liquid for <1 g
	  ○ 7.0 oz. liquid for ≥1 g
	• Consume the suspension
	• Resuspend residue in small amount of liquid and consume immediately
	• Tablets should not be chewed or swallowed whole
		• Once daily on an empty stomach or with a light meal (<7% fat; ~250 calories)
		• Swallow whole or crush and mix with soft foods such as yogurt or apple sauce immediately before use

Starting dose	• Transfusion-dependent iron overload: 20 mg/kg/day • NTDT: 10 mg/kg/day	• Transfusion-dependent iron overload: 14 mg/kg/day • NTDT: 7 mg/kg/day
Titration increments	• Transfusion-dependent iron overload: 5–10 mg/kg/day • NTDT: 5–10 mg/kg/day	• Transfusion-dependent iron overload: 3.5–7 mg/kg/day • NTDT: 3.5–7 mg/kg/day
Maximum dose	• Transfusion-dependent iron overload: 40 mg/kg/day • NTDT: 20 mg/kg/day	• Transfusion-dependent iron overload: 28 mg/kg/day • NTDT: 14 mg/kg/day

Table 2.
Deferasirox formulations: Key differences.

Author details

Tamer Hassan* and Marwa Zakaria
Department of Pediatric, Faculty of Medicine, Zagazig University, Zagazig, Egypt

*Address all correspondence to: dr.tamerhassan@yahoo.com

References

[1] Salehi R, Khosravi S, Salehi M, Kheirollahi M, Khanahmad H. Simple and easy to perform preimplantation genetic diagnosis for β-thalassemia major using combination of conventional and fluorescent polymerase chain reaction. Advanced Biomedical Research. 2017;**6**:23. DOI: 10.4103/2277-9175.201682

[2] Harper JC. Introduction. In: Harper JC, Delhanty JDA, Handyside AH, editors. Preimplantation Genetic Diagnosis. London, UK: John Wiley & Sons; 2001. pp. 3-12.

[3] Palmer GA, Traeger-Synodinos J, Davies S, et al. Pregnancies following blastocyst stage transfer in PGD cycles at risk for beta-thalassaemic haemoglobinopathies. Human Reproduction. 2002;**17**:25-31. DOI: 10.1093/humrep/17.1.25

[4] Thornhill AR, deDie-Smulders CE, Geraedts JP, et al. ESHRE PGD consortium best practice guidelines for clinical preimplantation genetic diagnosis (PGD) and preimplantation genetic screening (PGS). Human Reproduction. 2005;**20**:35-48. DOI: 10.1093/humrep/deh579

[5] Taher AT, Saliba AN. Iron overload in thalassemia: Different organs at different rates. Hematology. American Society of Hematology. Education Program. 2017;**2017**:265-271. DOI: 10.1182/asheducation-2017.1.265

[6] Sheth S. SQUID biosusceptometry in the measurement of hepatic iron. Pediatric Radiology. 2003;**33**:373-377. DOI: 10.1007/s00247-003-0877-x

[7] Srivastava A, Shaji RV. Cure for thalassemia major—From allogeneic hematopoietic stem cell transplantation to gene therapy. Haematologica. 2017;**102**:214-223. DOI: 10.3324/haematol.2015.141200

[8] Ferrari G, Cavazzana M, Mavilio F. Gene therapy approaches to hemoglobinopathies. Hematology/Oncology Clinics of North America. 2017;**31**:835-852. DOI: 10.1016/j.hoc.2017.06.010

[9] Karponi G, Zogas N. Gene therapy for beta-thalassemia: Updated perspectives. The Application of Clinical Genetics. 2019;**12**:167-180. DOI: 10.2147/TACG.S178546. eCollection 2019

[10] Makis A, Hatzimichael E, Papassotiriou L, Voskaridou E. 2017 clinical trials update in new treatments of β-thalassemia. American Journal of Hematology. 2016;**21**:1135-1145. DOI: 10.1002/ajh.24530

[11] Suragani RN, Cawley SM, Li R, et al. Modified activin receptor IIB ligand trap mitigates ineffective erythropoiesis and disease complications in murine β-thalassemia. Blood. 2014;**123**:3864-3872. DOI: 10.1182/blood-2013-06-511238

[12] Soni S. Novel and innovative approaches for treatment of β-thalassemia. Pediatric Hematology Oncology Journal. 2017;**2**:121-126. DOI: 10.1016/j.phoj.2017.11.153

[13] Blanchette NL, Manz DH, Torti FM, Torti SV. Modulation of hepcidin to treat iron deregulation: Potential clinical applications. Expert Review of Hematology. 2016;**9**:169-186. DOI: 10.1586/17474086.2016.1124757

[14] Saliba AN, Harb AR, Taher AT. Iron chelation therapy in transfusion-dependent thalassemia patients: Current strategies and future directions. Journal of Blood Medicine. 2015;**6**:197-209. DOI: 10.2147/JBM.S72463

[15] Novartis Pharmaceuticals. JADENU® (Deferasirox) US

Prescribing Information. 2015. Available from: www.pharma.us.novartis.com/product/pi/pdf/jadenu.pdf

[16] Perrine SP, Pace BS, Faller DV. Targeted fetal hemoglobin induction for treatment of beta hemoglobinopathies. Hematology/Oncology Clinics of North America. 2014;**28**:233-248. DOI: 10.1016/j.hoc.2013.11.009

[17] Angelucci E, Abutalib SA. Advances in transplantation and gene therapy in transfusion-dependent β-thalassemia. Advances in Cell and Gene Therapy. 2019;**2**:e25. DOI: 10.1002/acg2.25

Chapter 3

Transcriptional Repressors of Fetal Globin Genes as Novel Therapeutic Targets in Beta-Thalassemia

Marianna De Martino, Raffaele Sessa, Maria Rosaria Storino, Mariarosaria Giuliano, Silvia Trombetti, Rosa Catapano, Alessandra Lo Bianco, Paola Izzo and Michela Grosso

Abstract

During development the human β-globin gene cluster undergoes two *switching* processes at the embryo-fetal and fetal-adult stages, respectively, involving changes in chromatin remodeling and in transcriptional regulatory networks. In particular, during the perinatal period, the switch from fetal-to-adult globin gene expression leads to fetal globin genes silencing and progressive decline of fetal hemoglobin (HbF). Impaired hemoglobin switching is associated with hereditary persistence of HbF (HPFH), a condition in which the fetal globin genes fail to be completely silenced in adult red blood cells. This condition, when co-inherited with hemoglobinopathies, has great therapeutic potential because elevated HbF levels can ameliorate β-thalassemia and sickle cell anemia. Therefore, there is a growing interest about the complex network of factors that regulate fetal globin genes expression. Here we discuss the activity of transcriptional repressors of fetal globin genes and their potential role as novel therapeutic targets in β-thalassemia.

Keywords: globin gene switching, HbF silencing, LCR, transcriptional repressors, genome editing

1. Introduction

The human β-globin locus consists of five functional genes, *HBE*, *HBG2*, *HBG1*, *HBD*, and *HBB*, positioned on chromosome 11 in the same order in which they are expressed during ontogenesis. This fascinating process that regulates changes in the globin gene expression, referred to as *globin gene switching,* is programmed in order to produce different hemoglobin molecules able to meet the changing oxygen demand of the developing organism [1]. According to this process, up to the eighth week of pregnancy, the embryonic globin gene (*HBE*) is predominantly expressed in the primitive erythroblasts, large nucleated erythroid cells originating in the yolk sac. Approximately between the sixth and eighth week of pregnancy, fetal liver assumes the *hematopoietic role and produces small, enucleated erythroid cells*. The transition of hematopoiesis from the yolk sac to the fetal liver coincides with the switch from the embryonic *HBE* gene to the fetal globin genes (*HBG1* and *HBG2*). At the perinatal period, the *bone marrow becomes* the principal site of *hematopoiesis and generates mature* red blood *cells. In conjunction with the transition from* liver to bone marrow *hematopoiesis*, the second globin gene switch occurs from the fetal-to-adult globin genes (*HBD* and *HBB*) in which fetal hemoglobin (HbF) production gradually declines to be replaced by the adult type (HbA) [2].

In the last decades, large research efforts have been devoted to disclose the molecular mechanisms underlying this *switching* process, thus revealing how it is under the tight control of complex interactions involving dynamic changes in chromatin remodeling as well as in transcriptional regulatory networks. Nevertheless, it is rather common that residual amount of fetal globin genes continues to be expressed throughout adult life with the majority of adults having traces of HbF (approximately 1% of total hemoglobin). Impairment of this fetal-to-adult hemoglobin switching process, whose molecular basis has been associated with a heterogeneous group of inherited defects, leads to hereditary persistence of fetal hemoglobin (HPFH) in adult life. Based on clinical and genetic observations that HPFH has ameliorative effects in β-thalassemia and in sickle cell anemia (SCD), interest has been growing regarding the therapeutic potential of fetal globin gene reawakening for these disorders [3–5]. Therefore, much effort is currently underway in order to further clarify the molecular basis of hemoglobin switching and persistence of high HbF levels in adult life.

Fetal hemoglobin levels are regulated by complex mechanisms involving factors linked or not to the β-globin gene (*HBB*) locus. Several genetic determinants *in cis* to the *HBB* cluster, including large deletions in the *HBB* cluster or single nucleotide sequence variations in the regulatory regions of the fetal globin genes, are known to influence HbF levels [6, 7]. Also, HPFH quantitative trait loci (QTL) unlinked to the *HBB* cluster have been so far identified as being involved in the transcriptional control of fetal globin genes. In particular, in the last years, great attention has been focused on two genetic determinants, the *HBS1L-MYB* intergenic region located on chromosome 6q23 and the gene coding for the oncogenic transcriptional factor *BCL11A* on chromosome 2p16 that act as main QTLs in influencing HbF levels [8].

Below we discuss the contribution of some of the main cis- and trans-acting determinants so far identified in silencing fetal globin gene expression and the most recent therapeutic advances based on fetal globin gene reactivation in the treatment of hemoglobinopathies.

2. Regulatory elements and transcriptional factors involved in fetal globin gene silencing

2.1 The role of the locus control region (LCR) in chromatin remodeling and globin gene switching

The locus control region (LCR), located upstream of the *HBE* gene, represents the major regulatory element in the β-globin gene locus. It plays a key role in the switching process by controlling the transcription state of the locus as well as the transcription activity of each gene, thus conferring tissue- and stage-specific expression of the globin genes [9, 10].

The LCR contains five DNAse I hypersensitive sites (HS 1–5), four of which (HS1–HS4) acting as erythroid cell-specific enhancers that are required for proper order of activation of the globin genes during ontogeny. However, differently from classical enhancer elements, LCR activity is both orientation- and distance-dependent and prevents position effects, therefore also *indicating* an insulator function *for* this regulatory region [9]. The last hypersensitive site (HS5) has a different role, acting as a structural and insulator element. Indeed, in erythroid cells it is closely positioned to another hypersensitive site located at the opposite end of the *HBB* locus (3′HS1) to form an active chromatin hub that allows highly efficient globin gene transcription [10, 11].

It is now generally accepted that globin gene switching can occur through not mutually exclusive mechanisms involving direct competition between stage-specific gene promoters for LCR enhancer elements, gene expression activation, and/or silencing mechanisms promoted by specific activators and repressors as well as by epigenetic modifications. By chromatin conformation capture (3C) experiments, it has been shown that LCR exerts long-distance transcriptional enhancement through dynamic organization of the locus in stage-specific chromatin loops that allow the LCR enhancers to be positioned in close proximity of the genes that are to be activated [12]. This mechanism is also consistent with the evidence that the LCR can interact with only one promoter at a time. These interactions also strictly depend on the availability of specific trans-acting factors, non-DNA-binding factors linked to transcription factors and chromatin facilitators bound to regulatory regions of genes to be transcribed (**Figure 1**).

It has also been shown that epigenetic mechanisms at the *HBB* locus are involved in gene expression control. One of these mechanisms involves DNA and histone methylation processes that are generally associated with the repression state of globin genes in non-erythroid cells as well as with the erythroid stage-specific silencing of globin gene expression within the activated chromatin hub [13]. Recently, HS4 in LCR was found to regulate another important stage-specific epigenetic mechanism of gene expression control by contributing to drive the recruitment of different histone acetylation/deacetylation enzymatic activities at specific regulatory regions, with acetylation being a general hallmark of gene

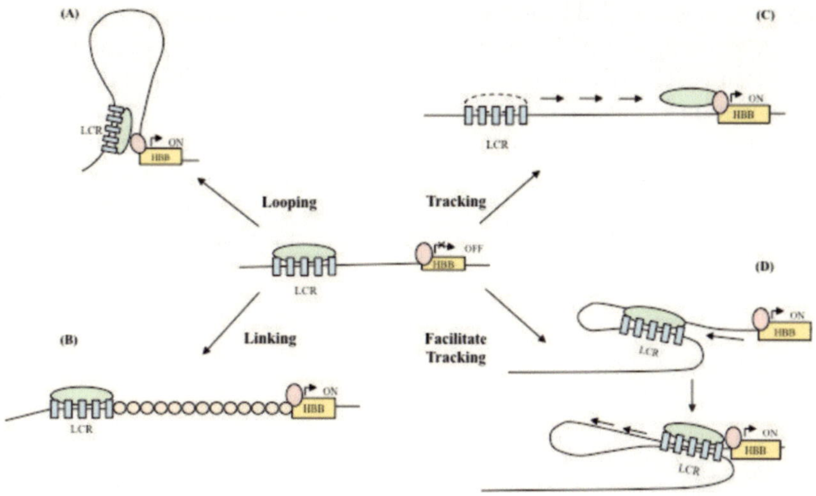

Figure 1.
Different molecular mechanisms proposed for LCR long-distance transcriptional enhancement through dynamic organization of the locus in stage-specific chromatin loops that allows the LCR enhances to be positioned in close proximity of the genes that are to be activated [9–12]. (A) The looping model is based on the concept that LCR acts as a holocomplex to stimulate gene expression by looping through the chromatin to activate the transcription machinery of a single gene at any given time. In this model, individual globin gene promoters are thought to compete for LCR activity. (B) The linking model requires the presence of a continuous protein chain from the LCR to the gene to be transcribed involving sequential stage-specific binding of transcriptional factors as well as of chromatin modifiers to define the chromatin region to be transcribed. (C) The tracking model is based on the idea that a signal such as an enhancer-bound protein complex comprising RNA polymerase II or histone modifiers is able to scan the DNA until a promoter is encountered to activate gene expression, with inactive genes looped out. (D) In the facilitated-tracking model, concepts of both the looping and tracking models are incorporated. In this model, enhancer-bound complexes track along DNA and, when the promoter of a to-be-transcribed gene is encountered, a stable DNA loop structure is formed.

activation and, on the contrary, deacetylation being associated with gene repression mechanisms. More recently, it has also been found that histone acetylation, besides activating high-level gene transcription, also contributes to the formation of specific chromatin looping leading to an open chromatin configuration at the *HBB* locus. Furthermore, it has also been proved that loss of histone acetylation increases methylation both in the LCR and in fetal globin genes, thus reinforcing the silencing mechanisms of these epigenetic modifications [11].

Chromatin looping, transcriptional protein complexes, and epigenetic modifications require a large array of protein factors whose list grows continuously, thus providing deeper insights into these mechanisms. The role of some of the most relevant of them will be herein discussed.

2.2 Cold-shock domain protein A (CSDA)

Cold-shock domain (CSD) proteins have been reported to be largely involved in a variety of gene expression regulation processes such as transcriptional activation and repression or posttranscriptional mechanisms including mRNA packaging, transport, localization, and stability. In these proteins the CSD domain does not bind to unique DNA sequence motifs, but it is able to recognize intramolecular triplex H-DNA structures, commonly generated by CT-rich sequences. The cold-shock domain protein A (CSDA), also known as DNA-binding protein A (dbpA), is a protein with a molecular weight of about 60 kDa [14]. The CSDA gene is located at position 12p13.1 and comprises 10 exons spanning a 24-kb genomic region. CSDA consists of three structural domains: an alanine/proline (AP)-rich N-terminal domain followed by a central cold-shock domain (CSD) and a C-terminal domain, containing four alternating clusters of basic and acid amino acids. The DNA-binding domain is encoded by exons 1–5. Within this region, the cold-shock domain, comprising about 70 amino acid residues, is encoded by exons 2–5 [14]. A RNP1 motif [GA] – [FY] – [GA] – [FY] – [IVA], conserved in this protein family [15], is present in the 3′ end of exon 2. The exon 6, encoding 69 amino acids, is alternatively spliced. The C-terminus (exons 6–9) C-terminal domain mediates protein-protein interactions [16]. Alternative splicing of exon 6 results in two main isoforms, namely, CSDA isoform *a* and isoform *b*, respectively, showing different C-terminal domains and thus potentially able to take part to specific protein complexes [14, 16].

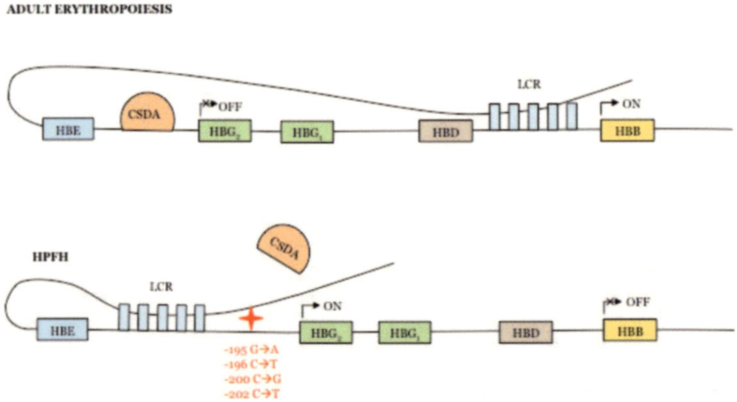

Figure 2.
Binding of the transcriptional repressor CSDA to the −200 promoter region of HBG2 *in adult erythropoiesis is impaired by HPFH mutations [18–22].*

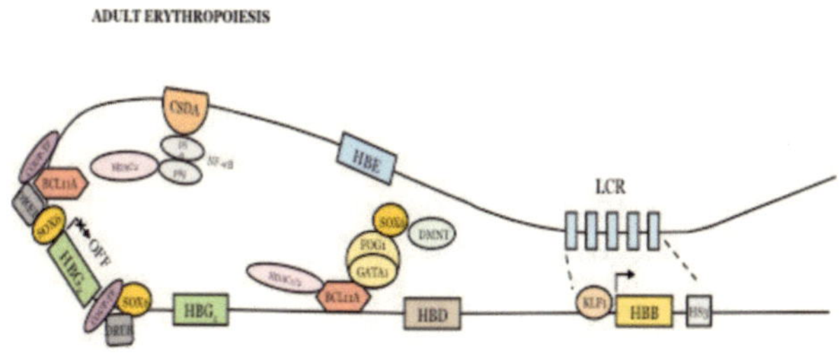

Figure 3.
Transcriptional repressor mechanisms of fetal globin genes in adult erythropoiesis involving BCL11A *and CSDA multiprotein complexes [23–27].*

CSDA *acts as a repressor of many cellular genes* including the human granulocyte-macrophage colony-stimulating factor (*GM-CSF*), an important hematopoietic growth factor [17]. More recently, it has been demonstrated that CSDA acts as a repressor of fetal globin gene expression by binding a region −200 bp upstream of the *HBG2* gene [18] (**Figure 2**). This region consists of alternating homopurine and homopyrimidine tracts generating an H-DNA structure [19]. Mutations (*HBG2* -200 C → G, −202 C → T, −196 C → T e − 195 G → A) that destabilize the intramolecular triplex structure have been found associated with HPFH [20]. Previous studies had suggested that disruption of the intramolecular triplex could abolish CSDA binding sites conditions in this *HBG2* promoter region [19, 21, 22], thus leading to persistent expression of fetal hemoglobin in adult life [19]. Based on RNA interference (RNAi) and overexpression studies in human erythroleukemia K562 cells and in primary erythroid cells, CSDA was demonstrated to directly play a repression role in *HBG* expression [18]. In fact, down- and up-modulation of CSDA levels consistently corresponded to variations of *HBG* expression levels: CSDA knockdown induced by RNAi resulted in significantly increased expression of HBG genes, whereas its overexpression was associated with reduced *HBG* mRNA levels. Also, chromatin immunoprecipitation (ChiP) analysis in K562 cells showed that CSDA interacts with this promoter region, thus confirming that CSDA modulates *HBG* expression at the transcriptional level [18]. Subsequently, it has been proposed that NF-kB and histone deacethylase 2 (HDAC2) interact with CSDA to form a multiprotein complex which take part to the regulation of *HBG2* expression by modulating local chromatin conformation [23], thus highlighting the relevance of the role played by CSDA in fetal globin gene expression and shedding novel light on the molecular mechanisms involved in globin gene switching (**Figure 3**).

2.3 B-cell lymphoma/leukemia 11A (BCL11A)

The *B-cell lymphoma/leukemia 11A* (BCL11A) is a multiple zinc-finger transcription factor encoded on chromosome 2p15, previously reported as being implicated in B-lymphocyte production and neurodevelopment [28]. More recently, genome-wide association studies (GWAS) identified single nucleotide polymorphisms (SNPs) in intron 2 of the *BCL11A* gene as strictly associated with HPFH conditions, thus revealing a hitherto unexplored but crucial role of *BCL11A in HbF silencing* [29]. *Indeed, as* was later demonstrated, such SNPs are able to disrupt erythroid-specific enhancer elements required for high-efficient expression of the *BCL11A gene* [30]. Similarly to CSDA, *BCL11A* knockdown experiments performed in K562 cells and in human erythroblasts led to increased expression of fetal globin genes, thus providing further evidence that this factor acts as a repressor of HbF expression.

In the last years, many efforts have been aimed at clarifying the repression mechanism exerted by BCL11A at the *HBB* locus. At this regard, an important contribution has been provided by the identification of the multiprotein complex interacting with BCL11A that includes GATA-1, FOG-1, RUNX1, KLF1, and SOX6 [24, 31, 32]. In addition, further insights have been provided regarding the BCL11A repression mechanisms by demonstrating how these protein complexes drive the recruitment of a variety of epigenetic factors such as the nucleosome remodeling and deacetylase (NuRD) repressor complex, histone deacetylase (HDAC1 and HDAC2), lysine-specific demethylase (LSD1), and DNA methyl-transferase (DNMT1) [25–27] (**Figure 3**). ChiP analysis also revealed binding sites for BCL11A at regulatory elements within the LCR, as well as at the promoter regions of both embryonic and fetal globin genes and in an intergenic region between the fetal and adult genes, thus indicating that these protein complexes are directly involved in fetal globin gene silencing as well as in long-range interactions that contribute to reshape chromatin loop domains in order to spatially separate the fetal and adult globin genes from the transcriptional machinery and, in the meantime, to promote long-range LCR interactions with the adult globin genes [33–35].

2.4 Krüppel-like factor 1 (KLF1)

The transcription factor KLF1 (Krüppel-like factor 1), formerly known as *erythroid Krüppel-like factor* (EKLF) for its restricted expression in erythroid cells and its similarity to the *protein* encoded by the *Drosophila* segmentation *Krüppel* gene), plays a multifunctional role in the regulation of a variety of cellular events leading to erythroid differentiation, including erythroid lineage commitment, heme synthesis, and globin gene switching [36–39].

The *KLF1* gene (~3kb) is located on chromosome region 19p13.2 and consists of three exons encoding a 362 amino acid protein with an N-terminal region rich in proline residues and containing two short transactivation domains (TAD1 and TAD2) and a C-terminus with three highly conserved Cys2/His2 zinc-finger domains (ZF1, ZF2, and ZF3) that interact with the DNA sequence motif 5′CCMCRCCCN3′ located in CACCC boxes and GC-rich elements in the regulatory regions of its target genes [38].

In the HBB cluster, KLF1 exerts a dual role in fetal-to-adult globin gene switching by different mechanisms. On one hand, as also evidenced by studies on (+/−) KLF1 transgenic mice [12], KLF1 contributes to directly activate the *HBB* gene in adult life by inducing the formation of chromatin loops that relieve the *HBB* gene from competition with the *HBG* genes and favor interactions of the HS2 and HS3 sites in the LCR with the *HBB* promoter region [40]. On the other hand, KLF1 indirectly contributes to silencing fetal globin gene expression through the activation of BCL11A, a repressor of *HBG* globin genes transcription, as described above. To date, more than 65 loss-of-function mutations have been reported for the *KLF1* gene, most of which are missense mutations found largely within the three zinc-finger domains [41]. Mutations in the *KLF1* gene have been reported to interfere with its functions in the erythropoiesis process, thus leading to a wide range of hematological phenotypes, including high borderline HbA2 levels, mild microcytosis, and/or hypochromia but also, importantly, with persistence of fetal hemoglobin expression in adult life. It is thus not surprising that, although identification of carriers of *KLF1* mutations may be quite challenging because their phenotypic traits do not present relevant clinical implications, the majority of *KLF1* mutations have been detected in populations at risk for hemoglobinopathies according to the evidence that defective KLF1 activity can lead to impaired HbF silencing with ameliorating effects in SCD and in β-thalassemia. Therefore, KLF1 mutations have been considered as a natural model of impaired hemoglobin switching, and, accordingly, KLF1 has been proposed as a new potential therapeutic target in these diseases [39, 42].

2.5 Myb

Myb is a DNA-binding transcriptional regulator of approximately 75 kDa that plays a crucial role in hematopoiesis and erythropoiesis. The *MYB* gene is located on chromosome 6q23 and codifies for a protein with three functional domains: a highly conserved DNA-binding domain (DBD) near its N-terminus that recognizes and binds the consensus sequence PyAACG/TG, a central transactivation domain (TAD), and a C-terminal negative regulatory domain (NRD) containing a leucine zipper motif important for *homodimeration* and for protein *interactions* [43].

A large variety of proteins have been identified so far as Myb interactors: DNA-binding transcription factors that directly bind Myb, transcriptional coactivators that mediate interactions with the transcriptional machinery, and protein factors that are able to modify Myb activity. Each of these of protein factors can act either as activator or repressor of Myb function, depending both on cell type and protein microenvironment [43].

In the last decade, a GWAS approach led to the identification of a set of single nucleotide polymorphisms at the *HBS1L-MYB* intergenic region, subsequently identified as *HMIP-2*, displaying a strong association with persistence of fetal hemoglobin in adult life [44–46]. By demonstrating that these SNPs disrupt binding sites at key erythroid enhancers and cause reduced Myb expression levels, it was possible to provide an explanation for the association of the HMIP-2 region with HbF levels and, in the meantime, to identify Myb as a negative regulator of fetal globin genes.

Notably, further evidence of the repressive role of Myb on fetal globin gene expression has also been provided by clinical observations of higher HbF levels in patients with trisomy 13. It has been demonstrated that in this condition, the high HbF levels are related to the dysregulation of two microRNAs, miR-15a and miR-16-1, both localized on chromosome 13q14, which mediate Myb downregulation through the binding to its 3′-UTR region [47].

Nevertheless, in spite of all these evidences, the mechanism of repression of fetal globin genes exerted by Myb is not fully understood. It has been proposed that Myb could regulate HbF expression by two not mutually exclusive mechanisms: by activating the expression levels of fetal globin gene repressors as BCL11A and KLF1 or by controlling the kinetics of erythroid differentiation. In fact, low Myb levels have been found associated with reduced levels of these *HBG* repressors and also with accelerated erythroid differentiation leading to the release of early erythroid progenitor cells that are still synthesizing predominantly HbF [48]. Furthermore, it has also been found that Myb and BCL11A cooperate with DNMT1 to achieve developmental repression of embryonic and fetal globin genes in adult erythropoiesis [25], thus supporting the evidence that the network of factors involved in fetal globin gene silencing converges on common mechanisms and cooperates at different levels to sustain *globin gene switching* and to reinforce the process of HbF repression.

3. Novel therapeutic approaches for β-thalassemia

Currently, clinical management of β-thalassemia and SCD patients is largely dependent on regular blood transfusions associated with chelating agents for the treatment of systemic iron overload. Indeed, except for allogeneic transplantation strategies, whose favorable outcome is anyway restricted to the availability of a well-matched donor, or for the more recent haploidentical transplantation option that however carries substantial risks, no other curative option is currently available for hemoglobinopathies. Therefore, due to the relevant global health burden of these diseases, there is still a great need for effective and definitive large-scale treatments.

In the last decades, given the ameliorative effects of elevated HbF levels that can lead to decreased hemoglobin polymerization in SCD as well as to reduced α-chain imbalance in β-thalassemia, a great deal of effort has been devoted to the development of new therapies aimed at reactivating fetal globin gene expression. Therefore, according to the evidences that hypo-methylated DNA and hyper-acetylated histones are well-known epigenetic marks of transcriptionally active regions, inhibitors of DNA methyltransferase (DNMT) and histone deacetylase (HDAC) have been developed as novel pharmacologic approaches to support transfusion therapy. Among the first drugs to be identified, 5-azacytidine and decitabine were found to induce increased HbF levels through DNA hypo-methylation process. Subsequently, the use of hydroxyurea (HU) was also investigated as a promising HbF inducer agent in adults with severe SCD. Although the mechanism through which HU induces HbF reactivation is still not completely understood, HU treatment was found to increase HbF levels and reduce HbS polymerization, thus improving clinical symptoms and quality of life of these patients. Another epigenetic approach was also exploited through the use of HDAC inhibitors, including butyrate and its derivatives that have been demonstrated to stimulate HbF production in β-thalassemia patients [49].

More recently, many hopes were directed toward the development of gene therapy procedures designed to introduce a normal copy of the β-globin gene by viral vectors that offer the advantages of long-term benefits and, even more importantly, being based on autologous transplant, do not require a matched donor. However, in spite of great expectations for a rapid development of this approach, for many years it proved a difficult goal, and only recently it has been successfully introduced in clinical practice. Notably, during the last years, additional promising therapeutic options have been provided by progress in gene-editing technologies, including the clustered, regularly interspaced, short palindromic repeat (CRISPR)-CRISPR-associated 9 (Cas9) (CRISPR-Cas9) tool, designed to introduce highly specific genome modifications for either gene disruption or correction [48, 50, 51]. At the same time, progress in understanding the molecular mechanisms underlying fetal globin gene silencing has contributed to identify several potential molecular targets, thus paving the way to novel therapeutic approaches for hemoglobinopathies that, besides correcting the defective β-globin gene, are now aimed at editing genomic segments that regulate fetal hemoglobin synthesis in hematopoietic stem cells (HSCs).

Interestingly, some of the most promising editing strategies for hemoglobinopathies that are being pursued include the reactivation of fetal globin genes that could be achieved either by silencing fetal globin gene repressors or, alternatively, by introducing known HPFH mutations in the HBB cluster. Since the beginning, targeting Myb or KLF1 appeared to be rather problematic given the pleiotropic roles played by these two factors in hematopoiesis and in erythropoiesis, respectively, whereas BCL11A emerged as one of the most appropriate candidate to be silenced, given its well-recognized role in HbF repression [48, 50, 51]. However, ubiquitous BCL11A knockdown rapidly turned out to be an unsuccessful strategy, given its role in other biological pathways including neuronal and B-lymphocyte development [28]. Consequently, alternative strategies are being underway focused on reducing its expression selectively in erythroid cells that could be achieved by disruption of its intronic erythroid-specific enhancer without affecting non-erythroid cells [51]. A similar approach could also be used to tune down Myb expression levels by editing SNPs at the *HBS1L-MYB* intergenic region that are known to disrupt the structure and the functionality of erythroid-specific enhancers causing reduced Myb expression levels. Anyway, other repressors such as CSDA or erythroid-specific cofactors could represent potential suitable candidates to be considered for novel genome-editing strategies. Furthermore, genome-editing procedures leading to the introduction of KLF1 mutations that emerged as a natural model of impaired hemoglobin switching or HPFH mutations in the regulatory regions of fetal globin genes have been proposed either as alternative or supportive therapeutic strategies to induce clinically significant increases in HbF levels [48, 50, 51].

4. Conclusions

The research in this field should be immediately focused on the development of safe, effective drug therapies that can be accomplished through fetal globin gene induction and at the same time on the prospect of cures through bone marrow transplantation using the promise of genome-editing strategies that will bring a vastly improved quality and quantity of life to patients who suffer from these devastating disorders.

Acknowledgements

This work was supported by the Regione Campania SATIN grant, grant/award number 2018–2020.

Conflict of interest

The authors declare no conflict of interest.

Author details

Marianna De Martino[1], Raffaele Sessa[1], Maria Rosaria Storino[1,2], Mariarosaria Giuliano[1], Silvia Trombetti[1], Rosa Catapano[1], Alessandra Lo Bianco[1], Paola Izzo[1,2] and Michela Grosso[1,2]*

1 Department of Molecular Medicine and Medical Biotechnology, University of Naples Federico II, Naples, Italy

2 CEINGE-Biotecnologie Avanzate, Naples, Italy

*Address all correspondence to: michela.grosso@unina.it

References

[1] Diepstraten ST, Hart AH. Modelling human haemoglobin switching. Blood Reviews. 2019;**33**:11-23. DOI: 10.1016/j.blre.2018.06.001

[2] Stamatoyannopoulos G. Control of globin gene expression during development and erythroid differentiation. Experimental Hematology. 2005;**33**(3):259-271. DOI: 10.1016/j.exphem.2004.11.007

[3] Cao A, Galanello R. Beta-thalassemia. Genetics in Medicine. 2010;**12**(2):61-76. DOI: 10.1097/GIM.0b013e3181cd68ed

[4] Akinsheye I, Alsultan A, Solovieff N, Ngo D, Baldwin CT, Sebastiani P, et al. Fetal hemoglobin in sickle cell anemia. Blood. 2011;**118**(1):19-27. DOI: 10.1182/blood-2011-03-325258

[5] Higgs DR, Engel JD, Stamatoyannopoulos G. Thalassaemia. Lancet. 2012;**379**(9813):373-383. DOI: 10.1016/S0140-6736(11)60283-3

[6] Dabke P, Colah RB, Ghosh K, Nadkarni A. Effect of a group of genetic markers around the 5′ regulatory regions of the β globin gene cluster linked to high HbF on the clinical severity of beta thalassemia. Blood Cells, Molecules & Diseases. 2013;**50**(3):156-160. DOI: 10.1016/j.bcmd.2012.11.003

[7] Menzel S, Thein SL. Genetic modifiers of fetal haemoglobin in sickle cell disease. Molecular Diagnosis & Therapy. 2019;**23**(2):235-244. DOI: 10.1007/s40291-018-0370-8

[8] Thein SL, Menzel S, Lathrop M, Garner C. Control of fetal hemoglobin: New insights emerging from genomics and clinical implications. Human Molecular Genetics. 2009;**18**(R2):R216-R223. DOI: 10.1093/hmg/ddp401

[9] Palstra RJ, de Laat W, Grosveld F. Beta-globin regulation and long-range interactions. Advances in Genetics. 2008;**61**:107-142. DOI: 10.1016/S0065-2660(07)00004-1

[10] Iarovaia OV, Kovina AP, Petrova NV, Razin SV, Ioudinkova ES, Vassetzky YS, et al. Genetic and epigenetic mechanisms of β-globin gene switching. Biochemistry. 2018;**83**(4):381-392. DOI: 10.1134/S0006297918040090

[11] Kim YW, Kim A. Histone acetylation contributes to chromatin looping between the locus control region and globin gene by influencing hypersensitive site formation. Biochimica et Biophysica Acta. 2013;**1829**(9):963-969. DOI: 10.1016/j.bbagrm.2013.04.006

[12] Noordermeer D, de Laat W. Joining the loops: β-globin gene regulation. IUBMB Life. 2008;**60**(12):824-833. DOI: 10.1002/iub.129

[13] Rank G, Cerruti L, Simpson RJ, Moritz RL, Jane SM, Zhao Q. Identification of a PRMT5-dependent repressor complex linked to silencing of human fetal globin gene expression. Blood. 2010;**116**(9):1585-1592. DOI: 10.1182/blood-2009-10-251116

[14] Kudo S, Mattei MG, Fukuda M. Characterization of the gene for dbpA, a family member of the nucleic-acid-binding proteins containing a cold-shock domain. European Journal of Biochemistry. 1995;**231**(1):72-82. DOI: 10.1111/j.1432-1033.1995.tb20672.x

[15] Landsman D. RNP-1, an RNA-binding motif is conserved in the DNA-binding cold shock domain. Nucleic Acids Research. 1992;**20**(11):2861-2864. DOI: 10.1093/nar/20.11.2861

[16] Kloks CP, Spronk CA, Lasonder E, Hoffmann A, Vuister GW, Grzesiek S,

et al. The solution structure and DNA-binding properties of the cold-shock domain of the human Y-box protein YB-1. Journal of Molecular Biology. 2002;**316**(2):317-326. DOI: 10.1006/jmbi.2001.5334

[17] Diamond P, Shannon MF, Vadas MA, Coles LS. Cold shock domain factor activate the granulocyte-macrophage colony-stimulating factor promoter in stimulated. The Journal of Biological Chemistry. 2001;**276**(11):7943-7951. DOI: 10.1074/jbc.M009836200

[18] Petruzzelli R, Gaudino S, Amendola G, Sessa R, Puzone S, Di Concilio R, et al. Role of the cold shock domain protein a in the transcriptional regulation of HBG expression. British Journal of Haematology. 2010;**150**(6):689-699. DOI: 10.1111/j.1365-2141.2010.08303.x

[19] Horwitz EM, Maloney KA, Ley TJ. A human protein containing a "cold shock" domain binds specifically to H-DNA upstream from the human γ-globin genes. The Journal of Biological Chemistry. 1994;**269**(19):14130-14139

[20] Coles LS, Diamond P, Occhiodoro F, Vadas MA, Shannon MF. Cold shock domain proteins repress transcription from the GM-CSF promoter. Nucleic Acids Research. 1996;**24**(12):2311-2317. DOI: 10.1093/nar/24.12.2311

[21] Bacolla A, Ulrich MJ, Larson JE, Ley TJ, Wells RD. An intramolecular triplex in the human γ-globin 5′-flanking region is altered by point mutations associated with hereditary persistence of fetal hemoglobin. The Journal of Biological Chemistry. 1995;**270**(41):24556-24563. DOI: 10.1074/jbc.270.41.24556

[22] Ulrich MJ, Gray WJ, Ley TJ. An intramolecular DNA triplex is disrupted by point mutations associated with hereditary persistence of fetal hemoglobin. The Journal of Biological Chemistry. 1992;**267**(26):18649-18658

[23] Gaudino S, Petruzzelli R, Amendola G, Sessa R, Puzone S, Risitano AM, et al. Structural and functional characterization of CSDA protein complexes involved in modulation of fetal globin gene expression. Blood. 2010;**116**(21):2071. DOI: 10.1182/blood.V116.21.2071.2071

[24] Xu J, Sankaran VG, Ni M, Menne TF, Puram RV, Kim W, et al. Transcriptional silencing of γ-globin by BCL11A involves long-range interactions and cooperation with SOX6. Genes & Development. 2010;**24**(8):783-798. DOI: 10.1101/gad.1897310

[25] Roosjen M, McColl B, Kao B, Gearing LJ, Blewitt ME, Vadolas J. Transcriptional regulators Myb and BCL11A interplay with DNA methyltransferase 1 in developmental silencing of embryonic and fetal beta-like globin genes. The FASEB Journal. 2014;**28**(4):1610-1620. DOI: 10.1096/fj.13-242669

[26] Rivers A, Vaitkus K, Ruiz MA, Ibanez V, Jagadeeswaran R, Kouznetsova T, et al. RN-1, a potent and selective LSD1 inhibitor, increases gamma-globin expression, F-retics, and F-cells in a sickle cell disease mouse model. Experimental Hematology. 2015;**43**(7):546-53.e1-3. DOI: 10.1016/j.exphem.2015.04.005

[27] Moody RR, Lo MC, Meagher JL, Lin CC, Stevers NO, Tinsley SL, et al. Probing the interaction between the histone methyltransferase/deacetylase subunit RBBP4/7 and the transcription factor BCL11A in epigenetic complexes. The Journal of Biological Chemistry. 2018;**293**(6):2125-2136. DOI: 10.1074/jbc.M117.811463

[28] Yu Y, Wang J, Khaled W, Burke S, Li P, Chen X, et al. Bcl11a is essential for lymphoid development and

negatively regulates p53. The Journal of Experimental Medicine. 2012;**209**(13):2467-2483. DOI: 10.1084/jem.20121846

[29] Sankaran VG, Menne TF, Xu J, Akie TE, Lettre G, Van Handel B, et al. Human fetal hemoglobin expression is regulated by the developmental stage-specific repressor BCL11A. Science. 2008;**322**(5909):1839-1842. DOI: 10.1126/science.1165409

[30] Funnell AP, Prontera P, Ottaviani V, Piccione M, Giambona A, Maggio A, et al. 2p15-p16.1 microdeletions encompassing and proximal to *BCL11A* are associated with elevated HbF in addition to neurologic impairment. Blood. 2015;**126**(1):89-93. DOI: 10.1182/blood-2015-04-638528

[31] Jawaid K, Wahlberg K, Thein SL, Best S. Binding patterns of BCL11A in the globin and GATA1 loci and characterization of the BCL11A fetal hemoglobin locus. Blood Cells, Molecules & Diseases. 2010;**45**(2):140-146. DOI: 10.1016/j.bcmd.2010.05.006

[32] Miccio A, Blobel GA. Role of the GATA-1/FOG-1/NuRD pathway in the expression of human beta-like globin genes. Molecular and Cellular Biology. 2010;**30**(14):3460-3470. DOI: 10.1128/MCB.00001-10

[33] Xu J, Bauer DE, Kerenyi MA, Vo TD, Hou S, Hsu YJ, et al. Corepressor-dependent silencing of fetal hemoglobin expression by BCL11A. Proceedings of the National Academy of Sciences of the United States of America. 2013;**110**(16):6518-6523. DOI: 10.1073/pnas.1303976110

[34] Martyn GE, Wienert B, Yang L, Shah M, Norton LJ, Burdach J, et al. Natural regulatory mutations elevate the fetal globin gene via disruption of BCL11A or ZBTB7A binding. Nature Genetics. 2018;**50**(4):498-503. DOI: 10.1038/s41588-018-0085-0

[35] Abdulazeez S. Molecular simulation studies on B-cell lymphoma/leukaemia 11A (BCL11A). American Journal of Translational Research. 2019;**11**(6):3689-3697

[36] Arnaud L, Saison C, Helias V, Lucien N, Steschenko D, Giarratana MC, et al. A dominant mutation in the gene encoding the erythroid transcription factor KLF1 causes a congenital dyserythropoietic anemia. American Journal of Human Genetics. 2010;**87**(5):721-727. DOI: 10.1016/j.ajhg.2010.10.010

[37] Borg J, Patrinos GP, Felice AE, Philipsen S. Erythroid phenotypes associated with *KLF1* mutations. Haematologica. 2011;**96**(5):635-638. DOI: 10.3324/haematol.2011.043265

[38] Perkins A, Xu X, Higgs DR, Patrinos GP, Arnaud L, Bieker JJ, et al. Krüppeling erythropoiesis: An unexpected broad spectrum of human red blood cell disorders due to KLF1 variants. Blood. 2016;**127**(15):1856-1862. DOI: 10.1182/blood-2016-01-694331

[39] Viprakasit V, Ekwattanakit S, Riolueang S, Chalaow N, Fisher C, Lower K, et al. Mutations in Kruppel-like factor 1 cause transfusion-dependent hemolytic anemia and persistence of embryonic globin gene expression. Blood. 2014;**123**(10):1586-1595. DOI: 10.1182/blood-2013-09-526087

[40] Deng W, Lee J, Wang H, Miller J, Reik A, Gregory PD, et al. Controlling long-range genomic interactions at a native locus by targeted tethering of a looping factor. Cell. 2012;**149**(6):1233-1244. DOI: 10.1016/j.cell.2012.03.051

[41] Liu D, Zhang X, Yu L, Cai R, Ma X, Zheng C, et al. KLF1 mutations are relatively more common in a thalassemia endemic region and ameliorate the severity of beta-thalassemia. Blood.

2014;**124**(5):803-811. DOI: 10.1182/blood-2014-03-561779

[42] Zhou D, Liu K, Sun CW, Pawlik KM, Townes TM. KLF1 regulates BCL11A expression and gamma- to beta-globin gene switching. Nature Genetics. 2010;**42**(9):742-744. DOI: 10.1038/ng.637

[43] Wang X, Angelis N, Thein SL. MYB-A regulatory factor in hematopoiesis. Gene. 2018;**665**:6-17. DOI: 10.1016/j.gene.2018.04.065

[44] Jiang J, Best S, Menzel S, Silver N, Lai MI, Surdulescu GL, et al. cMYB is involved in the regulation of fetal hemoglobin production in adults. Blood. 2006;**108**(3):1077-1083. DOI: 10.1182/blood-2006-01-008912

[45] Thein SL, Menze S, Peng X, Best S, Jiang J, Close J, et al. Intergenic variants of HBS1L-MYB are responsible for a major quantitative trait locus on chromosome 6q23 influencing fetal hemoglobin levels in adults. Proceedings of the National Academy of Sciences of the United States of America. 2007;**104**(27):11346-11351. DOI: 10.1073/pnas.0611393104

[46] Farrell JJ, Sherva RM, Chen Z, Luo H, Chu BF, Ha SY, et al. A 3-bp deletion in the HBS1L-MYB intergenic region on chromosome 6q23 is associated with HbF expression. Blood. 2011;**17**(18):4935-4945. DOI: 10.1182/blood-2010-11-317081

[47] Sankaran VG, Menne TF, Scepanovic D, Vergilio JA, Ji P, Kim J, et al. MicroRNA-15a and −16-1 act via MYB to elevate fetal hemoglobin expression in human trisomy 13. Proceedings of the National Academy of Sciences of the United States of America. 2011;**108**(4):1519-1524. DOI: 10.1073/pnas.1018384108

[48] Thein SL. Molecular basis of β thalassemia and potential therapeutic targets. Blood Cells, Molecules & Diseases. 2018;**70**:54-65. DOI: 10.1016/j.bcmd.2017.06.001

[49] Costa D, Capuano M, Sommese L, Napoli C. Impact of epigenetic mechanisms on therapeutic approaches of hemoglobinopathies. Blood Cells, Molecules & Diseases. 2015;**55**:95-100. DOI: 10.1016/j.bcmd.2015.05.004

[50] Lidonnici MR, Ferrari G. Gene therapy and gene editing strategies for hemoglobinopathies. Blood Cells, Molecules & Diseases. 2018;**70**:87-101. DOI: 10.1016/j.bcmd.2017.12.001

[51] Wienert B, Martyn G, Funnell APW, Quinlan KGR, Crossley M. Wake-up sleepy gene: Reactivating fetal globin for β-hemoglobinopathies. Trends in Genetics. 2018;**34**(12):927-940. DOI: 10.1016/j.tig.2018.09.004

Chapter 4

Nutraceutical Benefits of Green Tea in Beta-Thalassemia with Iron Overload

Pimpisid Koonyosying, Suthat Fucharoen and Somdet Srichairatanakool

Abstract

Secondary iron overload in patients with β-thalassemia is caused by multiple blood transfusions and increased iron absorption. Most of them die from cardiac arrest and infections while others from oxidative tissue damage and organ dysfunction. Under high saturation of transferrin with iron, redox-active iron such as non-transferrin-bound iron, labile plasma iron, and cellular labile iron pool is prone to the production of reactive oxygen species, oxidized biomolecules, oxidative tissue damages, and complications. Iron chelation therapy and antioxidant supplementation are a supportive treatment for patients' better quality of life and life expectancy. Green tea (*Camellia sinensis*) extract (GTE) is abundant with polyphenols, mainly epigallocatechin-3-gallate and nutraceuticals, which are beneficial for cell functions and health. Importantly, GTE possesses antioxidant, free radical scavenging, metal-chelating, anti-hemolysis properties in cell cultures, animals, and humans. This article has reported modes of actions and challenged such wonderful properties of green tea used to remove excessive iron, scavenge harmful radicals, restore malfunctions of vital organs, and treat patients with β-thalassemia with iron overload. Infeasibility and sustainability, the benefits of green tea can be applied for use in other diseases with iron toxicity and oxidative stress.

Keywords: *Camellia sinensis*, catechins, green tea, iron, oxidative stress, thalassemia

1. Introduction

Erythrocytes or red blood cells (RBC) play a crucial role in oxygen carrying and transportation. The main component of RBC is hemoglobin (Hb) which consists of four subunits of globin chain with heme group at the center of each subunit. The types of Hb can be defined by different globin chain compositions. For instances, hemoglobin A (HbA) consists of two α-globin chains and two β-globin chains ($\alpha_2\beta_2$), which is found in high levels of normal human blood. Hemoglobin A_2 (HbA_2) consists of two α-globin chains and two δ-globin chains ($\alpha_2\delta_2$), which is found in low levels of normal human blood and may be increased in the blood of patients with β-thalassemia. Fetal hemoglobin (HbF) consists of two α-globin chains and two γ-globin chains ($\alpha_2\gamma_2$), which is present in high levels in fetal and newborn human blood. Likewise, embryonic hemoglobin such as hemoglobin Gower I ($\zeta_2\varepsilon_2$) and Gower II ($\alpha_2\varepsilon_2$) are produced in early life and switched to other Hb types during development.

Human β-thalassemia is characterized by mutations of β-globin gene, resulting in deficient production of the β-globin chains of Hb molecule (ineffective erythropoiesis) and chronic anemia. Over 200 mutations have been identified in this gene, and the type of mutations can influence the severity of the disease. Blood transfusions aim to maintain normal Hb levels to prevent tissue hypoxia, whereas repeated blood transfusions lead to the inevitable consequence of iron accumulation in the body. Iron deposition occurs considerably in almost all tissues but is primarily located in the spleen, liver, heart, and endocrine glands. Besides ferritin iron and hemosiderin, the uncommon forms of iron including labile or transient iron pools (LIP) in the tissues, nonheme iron in RBC membrane, and non-transferrin-bound iron (NTBI) and labile iron pool (LPI) in plasma appear to be redox-active and subsequently generate reactive oxygen species (ROS) via Haber-Weiss and Fenton reactions. The ROS can oxidize biomolecules, causing oxidative tissue damage, organ dysfunctions, complications, and death. Effective iron chelation needs giving to counteract the resulting iron overload and prevent oxidative tissue damage. So far, monotherapy or combined therapy with iron chelators such as desferrioxamine (DFO), deferiprone (DFP), and deferasirox (DFX) has been used for the treatment of patients with β-thalassemia with iron overload, but they present some side effects. Modified medical regimens such as adjunctive iron chelator and antioxidant and drug cocktail are purported to increase the chelation efficacy, minimize the side effects, and achieve additive chelation efficacy. Moreover, commercially available antioxidants such as vitamin C, vitamin E, and *N*-acetylcysteine (NAC) are usually given together with the chelators to relieve the oxidative stress in patients with thalassemia. Herein, an interesting natural product such as green tea extract from tea leaves (*Camellia sinensis*) has been documented in terms of bifunctional antioxidant and iron-chelating properties in iron-overloaded cells and mouse and human thalassemia, rather than its general biological and pharmacological properties.

2. β-Thalassemia

2.1 Etiology and pathophysiology

β-Thalassemia is a quantitative hemoglobinopathy which impairs the production of β-globin chains in Hb due to mutations of the gene located on the short arm of chromosome 11. Accordingly, a reduction of β^+ or an absence of β^0 in β-globin synthesis causes the precipitation of excessive unbound α-globin chains in erythroid precursors due to chain imbalances. The abnormal erythroid precursors are driven into apoptosis pathway during their differentiation and maturation in the bone marrow, consequently leading to erythroid expansion, accelerated extramedullary erythropoiesis, increased dietary iron absorption, and high turnover of RBC. Moreover, impaired β-globin synthesis and ineffective erythropoiesis result in microcytic anemia and progressive splenomegaly. There are three main types of β-thalassemia, in order of decreasing severity, homozygous β-thalassemia major (TM), β-thalassemia intermedia (TI), and heterozygous β-thalassemia minor. Hemoglobin E (HbE)/β-thalassemia is the most prevalent in Southeast Asia where the carrier frequency is around 50%. The interaction of HbE and β-thalassemia results in a clinical spectrum ranging from a severe condition that is indistinguishable from TM to a mild form of TI [1].

Nowadays, β-thalassemia is divided into transfusion-dependent β-thalassemia (TDT) and non-transfusion-dependent β-thalassemia (NTDT). In other mammals, mouse homozygous beta-globin knockout (BKO) thalassemia shows many clinical features of abnormal RBC indices including a decrease in blood Hb concentration, hematocrit (Hct), RBC numbers, and osmotic fragility and an increase of reticulocyte count. Likely, increased degradation of abnormal RBC is an important consequence of unstable Hb and excessive membrane iron in patients with β-thalassemia. Invasive and noninvasive laboratory investigations reveal systemic and cellular iron overload in TDT and NTDT patients. Large amounts of the irons from enterocytes and reticuloendothelial (RE) macrophages in the spleen can get into plasma compartment and subsequently bind to transferrin (Tf). Accordingly, this can lead to a high saturation of Tf with iron, an appearance of NTBI and LPI, and high levels of ferritin in plasma compartment, together with high iron deposition ferritin (Ft) in several tissues in the body. Consequently, iron accumulation in the vital organs is the cause of susceptibility to infections and immunological abnormalities, liver diseases (e.g., hepatitis, hepatic fibrosis, and hepatocellular carcinoma), cardiomyopathies (e.g., cardiac arrhythmia and heart failure), and endocrine gland dysfunction (e.g., diabetes, growth retardation, hypogonadism, and hypoparathyroidism) [2–4]. Evidentially, most of patients with β-thalassemia with iron overload die of heart failure, while some patients frequently die from infections and suffer from liver diseases and endocrinopathies.

2.2 Iron overload and oxidative stress

2.2.1 Iron transport into cells

In fact, abnormal iron absorption in patients with thalassemia produces an increase in the body iron burden evaluated at 2–5 g per year, and regular blood transfusion (420 mL/U, equivalent to 200 mg of iron) leads to double iron accumulation [5]. Normally, iron is bound to iron-transporting protein in plasma (called transferrin) and in milk (called lactoferrin), forms transferrin-bound iron (TBI), and is transported in blood circulation to target cells. The circulating TBI, which is low saturation in iron-deficiency persons, one-third saturation in normal people, and high saturation in iron overload patients, is taken up into iron-requiring target cells by using ATP-dependent transferrin receptor 1 (TfR1)-mediated endocytosis and delivered in cells for functions and storage in ferritin molecules (H- and L-subunits). When the capacity of transferrin to incorporate iron derived from gastrointestinal (GI) tract and RE cells becomes limited, the transferrin iron-binding capacity (TIBC) has been surpassed [6]. Afterward, two forms of redox-active iron such as NTBI and LPI appear primarily in plasma of patients with β-thalassemia. Pathologically, the NTBI fraction seems to translocate across plasma membrane via specific transporters on specific cell types. NTBI transporter which is originally called divalent metal ion transporter 1 (DMT1) or natural resistance-associated macrophage protein 2 (Nramp2) is proposed to locate on intestinal epithelial cells, erythroid cells and astrocytes, L-type calcium channel (LTCC), T-type calcium channel (TTCC) on cardiomyocytes, T-type calcium channel (TTCC) on hepatocytes, pancreatic islets β cells and kidney tubular cells, anion-exchange protein 2 (AE2) on bronchial epithelial cells, ferrireductases on kidney proximal tubule, and zinc ion protein 18 (ZIP18) on kidney tubular cells and hippocampal neuronal cells [7–14]. Importantly, NTBI and LPI are redox-active and susceptible to chelation [15].

2.2.2 Iron overload

The iron that cells do not require immediately for metabolic processes is stored in ferritin in the liver, enterocytes, and RE macrophages, representing the storage iron pool. The iron that mobilizes transiently inside the cells is called LIP that is potentially redox-active and increased when the cells are heavily loaded with a large number of extracellular irons, TBI, and NTBI. Iron distribution in the body is strictly regulated by two regulatory systems, systemic and cellular iron homeostasis. Systemic iron homeostasis strictly responds to ensure a balance of iron absorption and iron utilization, which relies on the hepatic hepcidin hormone and the ferroportin actions and occurs in enterocytes, hepatocytes, and splenic macrophages. Hepcidin levels found to decrease in primary hemochromatosis and secondary hemochromatosis such as TI patients due to an acceleration of erythropoietic activity driven by increases of erythropoietin (EPO) production and TfR1 expression. Inversely, hepcidin levels increased in TM patients due to blood transfusion that they do not need to increase erythropoiesis to compensate ineffective erythropoiesis [16]. The regulation will reduce iron efflux from ferroportin at the basolateral part of duodenal epithelial cells and from RE macrophage into the plasma, resulting in iron retention within the cells. Drugs or natural products that increase hepcidin expression and production would be beneficial for the supportive treatment of TI patients with iron overload. Cellular iron homeostasis is dependent on the expression and function of TfR1 and ferritin mediated by iron regulatory element (IRE)/iron regulatory protein (IRP) system. Once TBI is internalized into cells via TfR-mediated endocytosis, iron is mainly stored by ferritin inside the cells [17]. In patients with thalassemia, large amounts of iron from diet and degradation of effete RBC by RE macrophage drain into plasma transferrin and subsequently taken into cells. Consequently, this will result in iron overload, oxidative stress, and depletion of antioxidant defense systems in plasma compartment and many vital organs in the body.

2.2.2.1 Blood

Thalassemia RBC containing large amounts of iron and low protective antioxidant system is prone to be damaged by ROS, leading to chronic hemolytic anemia. In young patients with β-thalassemia, plasma and RBC levels of thiobarbituric acid-reactive substances (TBARS), superoxide dismutase (SOD), and ferritin were increased, but the level of catalase (CAT) was decreased when compared with normal children [18]. Interestingly, Aphinives and colleagues have found decreased levels of antioxidants such as reduced glutathione (GSH) and vascular endothelial dysfunction in young Thai patients with β-thalassemia with HbE patients [19]. Additionally, blood levels of CAT, glutathione-*S*-transferase (GST), GSH, and vitamin C were found to decrease in β-thalassemia major patients while blood SOD level was increased [20]. Importantly, the levels of blood antioxidant system including GST, glutathione peroxidase (GPx), glutathione reductase (GR), peroxiredoxin 2 (Prx2), thioredoxin 1, and thioredoxin reductase were decreased in β-thalassemia major patients with regular blood transfusion and iron chelation therapy, whereas the blood levels of CAT and SOD were increased when compared to healthy subjects [21]. Consistently, the levels of red cell SOD, GPx, and CAT activities increased in hemoglobin H (HbH) disease (a moderately severe α-thalassemia) patients when compared to healthy control. However, the Chinese medicine "Yisui Shengxue" granules which have been officially prescribed and clinically used for the treatment of thalassemia for a long time effectively decreased the GPx and CAT activities but increased the SOD activity [22]. Prolonged bleeding times and abnormal platelet aggregation can be found in transfusion-dependent β-thalassemia major patients, possibly due to artifacts caused by in vitro manipulations, oxidative platelets, and circulating procoagulants such as microparticles (MP) tissue factors and platelet-derived MP [23, 24]. Platelet numbers were approximately 1.5- and 4-fold increase in Thai non-splenectomized and splenectomized patients with HbE/β-thalassemia when compared with normal subjects [25]. In comparison, thrombocytosis, platelet hyperaggregation, and decreased levels of protein S, protein C, and antithrombin III were detected in NTDT (such as TI) patients (9.4% with splenectomy and 90.6% without splenectomy) [26]. Increased oxidative stress of thalassemia platelets was restored by the treatment of iron chelators such as DFO and antioxidants such as NAC and vitamin C [24].

2.2.2.2 Spleen

The spleen is an organ containing some of the RE cells that function to destroy RBC hemoglobin by macrophages and store the released iron in the form of ferritin and hemosiderin. The number of blood transfusions in β-thalassemia major patients seems to correlate with their splenic hemosiderosis and splenic weight [27]. Hemosiderin deposition was found to be greater in the iron-overloaded livers than in the iron-overloaded spleens. Ferritin and hemosiderin increased in hepatocytes and splenic RE cells [28]. Splenectomy is one of the therapeutic options in hyper-transfused β-thalassemia major patients to reduce hyperactivity of RE macrophages; nevertheless, it may increase the iron overload. As a consequence, complications in patients with splenectomized thalassemia have included hypercoagulability, an increased incidence of vascular thrombosis, and an increased risk of infection. Iron overload in the spleen can activate latent nuclear factor-kappa B (NFκB) in alveolar macrophage, reduce immunity, and increase susceptibility to infection [29]. Notably, Prx2, which is a typical-2 cysteine peroxiredoxin and a key antioxidant system, is upregulated during erythropoiesis in patients with β-thalassemia and contributes to the stress erythropoiesis in the patients. Nuclear factor erythroid 2 (Nrf2) is a redox-response transcriptional nuclear factor and cellular adaptive process in response to and protection of oxidative stress [30]. Therefore, the regulation of *Prx2* and *Nrf2* genes results in the upregulation of antioxidant (antioxidant responsive element, ARE) genes required to ensure the survival of iron-overloaded cells.

2.2.2.3 Liver

The liver is one of the main storage organs for iron. Iron overload is considered to be when the ferritin level consistently exceeds 1000 ng/mL (normal range 20–200 ng/mL). Excess free radicals can cause progressive tissue injury and eventually cirrhosis or hepatocellular carcinoma in iron overload patients whose iron is sequestrated predominantly in ferritin or hemosiderin [31]. When plasma transferrin becomes highly saturated, NTBI is detectable and is rapidly transported across the hepatocyte membrane via a specific pathway. Likely, ferroportin 1 is the only protein that mediates the transport of iron out of hepatocytes and is then oxidized by ceruloplasmin and bound to transferrin. Iron deposition affects hepatic parenchymal cells (hepatocytes and bile duct cells) and mesenchymal cells (endothelial cells, macrophage, and Kupffer cells) and often distributes differently from one area to another [32]. As mentioned above, iron overload can induce ROS which can oxidize biomolecules. Lipid peroxidation activates tumor growth factor-beta1 (TGF-β1) expression which is the most potent pro-fibrogenic cytokine, and its expression is increased in almost all of fibrotic diseases. Type I collagen is induced by TGFβ resulting in uncontrolled collagen production and leads to tissue scarring and organ failure. The scar tissue replaces normal parenchyma, increases fibrosis, and blocks the liver portal blood flow consequently generating liver cirrhosis.

2.2.2.4 Heart

Iron overload cardiomyopathy is a common cause of death in patients with β-thalassemia. Biochemically, irons in iron-sulfur clusters and cytochromes are key players for oxidative phosphorylation and superoxide production in the mitochondria. Iron deposition in the heart cells seems to lead oxidative stress and cellular damage. The heart is the most mitochondrial-rich tissue in the body, making iron of particular importance to cardiac function. In cardiac cells, excess iron may result in oxidative stress and alteration of myocardial function because of the DNA damage caused by hydrogen peroxide through the Fenton reaction. Heart failure is the leading cause of death among patients with β-thalassemia with hemosiderosis, of whom around 60% die from cardiac failure. Harmful effects of iron overload on the heart of β-thalassemia major patients can be monitored using noninvasive and invasive techniques. Treatment with iron chelators can protect these patients from cardiac disease induced by iron overload [33–36].

2.2.2.5 Bone marrow

Bone marrow iron deposition (186 μg/g wet weight) increases in proportion to the total body iron stored in a dietary iron overload of African Bantu people and Caucasian patients with idiopathic hemochromatosis [37]. Myelodysplastic syndrome patients who are a heterogeneous group of clonal hematopoietic stem cell malignancies show bone marrow hemosiderosis and also develop systemic iron overload.

2.2.2.6 Endocrine glands

Though hematologic care has improved in patients with homozygous transfusion-dependent β-thalassemia, multi-endocrine dysfunction is still a common complication. Thyroid dysfunction defined as overt hypothyroidism, subclinical hypothyroidism, and exaggerated thyroid-stimulating hormone response was reported in patients with β-thalassemia [38]. In addition, lower serum thyroxine and higher thyrotrophic hormone levels were found in young patients with thalassemia than in normal children. Pituitary siderosis of β-thalassemia major patients causes oxidative tissue damage [39], consequently hypogonadotropic hypogonadism and growth hormone deficiency. Approximately half of the patients' pituitary gland dysfunction associated with iron overload is irreversible. Toxic irons in patients with β-thalassemia major (TDT) and patients with HbE/β-thalassemia are catalytically harmful to adrenal glands and can cause adrenal function insufficiency [40]. A previous study demonstrated that all β-thalassemia major patients were nondiabetic and some of them have decreased oral glucose tolerance test. They showed a normal response of cortisol to insulin and adrenocorticotropic hormone stimulation [41]. Moreover, the β cell pancreatic function and adrenal cortical function are depressed in severe iron loaded. The pancreas is another vital organ for iron accumulation especially pancreatic β cell in the islet of Langerhans. Importantly, TDT patients present iron deposition in the pancreatic beta cells beginning in the early age of life, resulting in decreased insulin secretion [42]. Normal iron level mediates insulin secretion via electron transport chain and endoplasmic reticulum calcium release by ROS triggering. Inversely, highly accumulated iron produces a high level of ROS which damages cell organelles and consequently affects iron-mediated insulin secretion mechanism (**Figure 1**).

As mentioned above, iron overload in thalassemia was assessed with a highly elevated level of plasma iron, and highly accumulated tissue iron concentrations

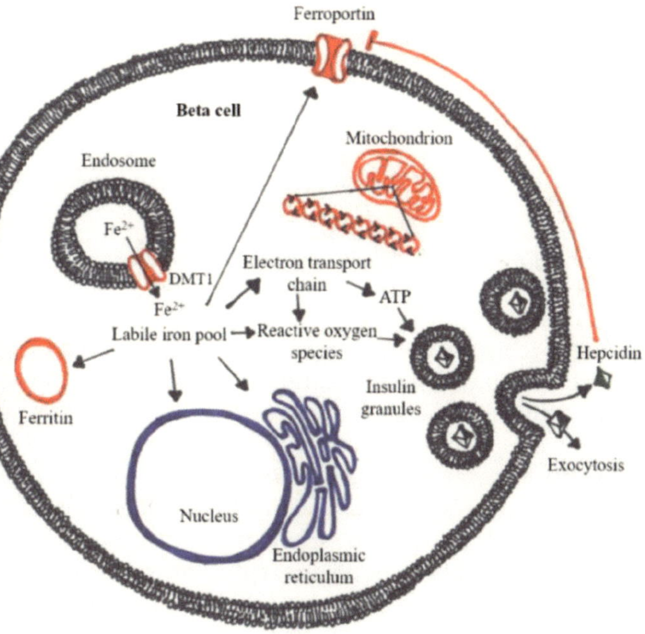

Figure 1.
Iron-mediated insulin secretion in pancreatic β cells (modified from [42]). Abbreviations/symbols: ATP = adenosine-5′-triphosphate, DMT1 = divalent metal ion transporter 1, Fe^{2+} = ferrous ion.

lead to many complications. Importantly, effective iron chelators are regularly administrated to patients with β-thalassemia for removing the redox iron, ameliorating the complications, and prolonging their life expectancy.

2.2.3 Oxidative stress

Iron can participate in the redox process known as the Haber-Weiss/Fenton reactions to generate ROS including hydrogen peroxide (H_2O_2) and hydroxyl radical ($OH^•$) (**Figure 2**) [43]. Subsequently, ROS can oxidize biomolecules such as proteins, carbohydrates, lipids, and nucleic acids in the body causing oxidative tissue damage, organ dysfunctions, complications, and pathogenesis [44, 45]. In addition, ROS can induce cell apoptosis through initiating serial chemical reactions including DNA strand breakage and fragmentation, protein oxidation, and lipids peroxidation [43, 46, 47]. Excessive redox iron can also react with unsaturated lipids to produce alkoxyl and peroxyl radicals [48]. These oxidative reactions result in the impairment of cellular functions and lead to damage of cells, tissues, and organs, which is evident in the iron-loading diseases, β-thalassemia, and Friedreich's ataxia.

2.3 Assessment methods

For blood samples, the levels of serum iron, TIBC, transferrin saturation, ferritin, soluble transferrin receptors, protoporphyrin IX, and routinely measured iron parameters indicate whether the body iron status is normal iron balance, iron deficiency, or iron overloaded. In addition, the levels of redox irons (e.g., NTBI and LPI) and iron-responsive proteins such as EPO, hepcidin, and erythroferrone (ERFE) are determined to distinguish the iron imbalance.

Biopsied liver tissue is a clinical sample that is collected for stoichiometric determination of nonheme iron. However, this invasive technique requires an

$$Fe^{2+} + O_2 \rightarrow Fe^{3+} + O_2^{\bullet-} \qquad \textbf{Haber-Weiss reaction}$$

$$O_2^{\bullet-} + 2H^+ \xrightarrow{SOD} H_2O_2$$

$$Fe^{2+} + H_2O_2 \rightarrow Fe^{3+} + HO^- + HO^\bullet \qquad \textbf{Fenton reaction}$$

Figure 2.
Iron-catalyzed generation of reactive oxygen species. Abbreviations/symbols: Fe^{2+} = ferrous ion, Fe^{3+} = ferric ion, SOD = superoxide dismutase.

expert hepatologist to operate. The liver tissue will be investigated for its iron content using histochemical Pearl's staining, physical atomic absorption spectrometry (AAS), and colorimetric ferrozine methods. Liver iron concentration (LIC) is correlated closely with serum ferritin concentration and is a valuable alternative to assess visceral iron overload in heavily iron-loaded β-thalassemia major patients. In contrast, the collection of other tissues such as the myocardium, liver, pancreas, adrenal glands, anterior pituitary gland, and skin would be too harmful to be collected [49]. Sophisticated noninvasive techniques including magnetic resonance imaging [50], magnetic iron detector susceptometry, superconducting quantum interference device, and nuclear resonance scattering are used to assess iron content in tissues. These methods are valuable for evaluating iron load in the tissues and monitoring the response of different organs to chelation therapy.

2.4 Iron chelation therapy

Iron chelation therapy aims to prevent the accumulation of toxic iron and eliminate the excess iron in patients with transfusion-dependent β-thalassemia. Effective chelation and good management of the patients have correlated with a decline in early deaths and complications. The reduction of plasma and cellular chelatable irons (e.g., NTBI, LPI, and LIP) is a slow process and requires aggressive chelation therapy. The chelation will maintain the iron balance at safe levels to prevent high iron accumulation and oxidative tissue injury. Such non-iron and iron-overloaded models as RBC, cell cultures (e.g., hepatocytes, HepG2 cells, and cardiomyocytes), animals (e.g. mice, gerbils, rats, and transgenic BKO mice), and even human patients with thalassemia are experimentally investigated and clinically tested to assess the safety and efficacy of various iron chelators. Individually, DFO, DFP, and DFX are promising iron chelators widely used for the treatment of patients with β-thalassemia with iron overload. Combined DFO/DFP and DFP/DFX treatments can reverse endocrine complications by improving glucose intolerance and gonadal dysfunction in TD-TM patients [51].

A combination therapy is when two chelators were combined and presented some degree of overlap which pharmacologically lead to improve efficacy and rate of iron removal [52–54]. The most extensively studied combination therapy is a combination between DFO and the oral chelator DFP which has been shown to rapidly reduce liver iron, serum ferritin, and myocardial siderosis compared with DFO monotherapy. Clinical trial data for the combination of DFX and DFO chelation has reinforced the benefits of combination therapy [55]. In addition, the clinical combination of DFX and DFP would be more appealing to patients than other combination therapy regimens involving the parenterally administered DFO. However, concrete data regarding the safety, efficacy, and dosing of each regimen are limited.

In principle, when two chelators are used together, they can act either additively or synergistically. Additivity refers to the predicted level of effect achieved by a drug combination based on individual drug potencies, whereas synergy refers to the exaggerated effect noted upon concurrent use of drugs. Synergism may occur in conditions allowing "iron shuttling." The rate of the chelators' access to cells, both in vitro and in vivo, is determined by size, charge, and lipid solubility of the chelators [55–58]. In plasma, the previous demonstration showed that low concentrations of DFP can act as a "shuttle" by gaining more rapid access to some non-transferrin-bound iron (NTBI) pools than DFO and subsequently donating iron to a DFO as a "sink" [54]. The isobologram analysis was reported to distinguish between synergistic, additive, or a sub-additive response to iron chelator combinations in human hepatic cells (HuH7) [59]. The synergy can imply that the primary chelator can act as a "shuttle" for iron chelated and delivered to the secondary "sink" chelator at low concentrations (**Figure 3**).

2.5 Supplementation of antioxidants

All patients with β-thalassemia have higher oxidative stress levels than normal people. Hitherto, supplementation of antioxidants has been recommended for them to ameliorate oxidative stress, give a better quality of life, and sustain long lives. Many antioxidants such as water-soluble vitamins C (L-ascorbic acid), fat-soluble vitamin E (α-tocopherol), and vitamin A, β-carotenoids, glutathione, curcuminoids, and quercetin are the compounds of interest.

2.5.1 Vitamin C

The levels of AA in leukocytes, platelets, and urine of patients with iron overload such as patients with idiopathic hemochromatosis, TDT patient, and Bantu people were decreased [60, 61]. After treatment of TM patients with AA, the serum levels of iron, transferrin saturation, and ferritin were increased [62]. Possibly, AA would involve mobilization of storage iron from tissue ferritin by reducing ferric oxyhydroxide to ferrous ion, which will subsequently catalyze ROS production via Haber-Weiss reaction and increase oxidative damage in the patients. However,

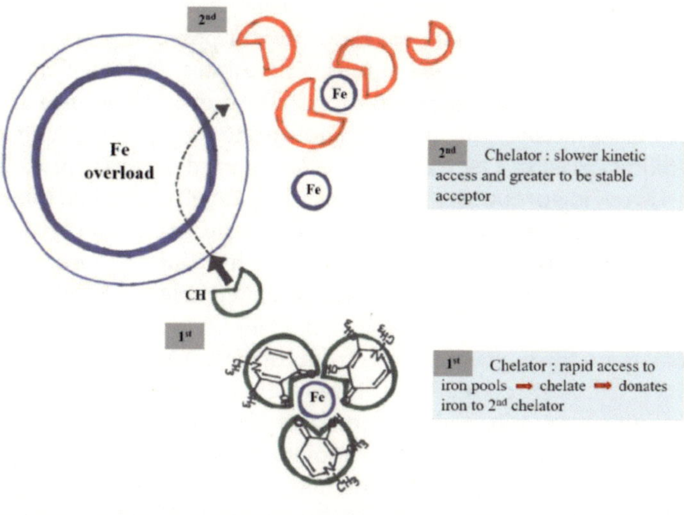

Figure 3.
Iron shuttling mechanism described combination therapy. Abbreviations/symbol: CH = chelator, Fe = iron.

vitamin C plus vitamin E supplementation seemed to be more effective than vitamin E alone for promoting antioxidant activity in patients with β-thalassemia [63].

2.5.2 Vitamin E

Evidently, the serum levels of vitamins A, vitamin E, zinc, selenium, and copper were decreased in young patients with thalassemia, while the serum levels of retinol and selenium inversely correlated with those of iron and ferritin. Moreover, low serum level of vitamin E was found in homozygous β-thalassemia and β-thalassemia/Hb E. Administration of vitamin E and polyphenols together with iron chelators abolished the increase of oxidative stress in patients with thalassemia, suggesting a substantial improvement of their anemia and complications [64]. The results from clinical studies using curcuminoids and vitamin E supported the free radical scavenging activity in the improvement of oxidative stress and platelet functions in patients with thalassemia [65, 66]. Surprisingly, oral administration of high doses of vitamin E effectively decreased plasma lipid peroxidation in patients with β-thalassemia and prolonged RBC survival in some patients. Furthermore, the treatment of TM and TI patients with vitamin E (750 to 1000 IU/day) for 16 months showed a fourfold increase in serum and RBC vitamin E levels and a reduction of serum malondialdehyde (MDA) level when compared with the untreated group [41]. Unchern and colleagues have reported that daily vitamin E supplementation for 3 months significantly increased plasma β-tocopherol levels and decreased plasma oxidant levels in splenectomized β-thalassemia/Hb E patients [66].

2.5.3 N-Acetylcysteine

NAC is a potent antioxidant and free radical scavenger, which involves glutathione biosynthesis and promotes detoxification. It is utilized for the treatment option for sickle cell anemia and diseases involved in the generation of ROS. Under iron overload condition, NAC provides a protective effect on brain dysfunction in iron-overloaded rats; therefore, the compound can diminish ROS production and DNA damage in patients with β-thalassemia [67–69].

2.5.4 Natural products

Quercetin is one of the predominant flavonoids of polyphenolics found in many fruits, vegetables, leaves, grains, red onions, kale, apples, and tea. Flavonoids are commonly present in their glycosylated form in the diet and presence of aglycone, glycoside, as well as methyl, glucuronide, and sulfate conjugates, which have been reported in human plasma. Quercetin has been reported to exert antioxidant and free radical scavenging properties in vitro, while quercetin supplementation has been promoted for the treatment of cancer and other diseases. Surprisingly, dietary quercetin supplementation was found to attenuate liver injury in iron-overloaded mice [70]. As a novel idea, we wish to investigate their role as adjuncts in iron mobilization [71].

Curcuminoids are the phytochemicals from turmeric *Curcuma longa* Linn (family Zingiberaceae), which are composed of three main constituents including curcumin, demethoxycurcumin, and *bis*-demethoxycurcumin, in which the important bioactive molecular structure is diketone moiety. Curcumin was found to suppress the ROS generation and lipid peroxidation in erythrocytes. Surprisingly, curcumin metabolites including di-, tetra-, and hexa-hydrocurcumin exhibit strong antioxidant, free radical scavenging, anti-lipid peroxidative and iron-chelating properties. The other effects are antithrombotic and anti-inflammatory activities. Oxidative stress condition in red blood cells of β-thalassemia/HbE patients is reduced after treatment with curcuminoids [65], leading to an improvement of their quality of life.

Green tea exhibits many interesting biological, biochemical, and pharmacological properties in health benefits. Normally, tea leaves (*Camellia sinensis*) are processed without fermentation for the preparation of green tea extract (GTE), which is abundant with epigallocatechin-3-gallate (EGCG) and exhibits antioxidative iron-chelating activity. In a recent study, the effect of GTE products on the status of iron overload, oxidative stress, and endocrine hormones was studied in iron overload pancreatic and liver cell lines, β-thalassemic mice, and β-thalassemia/HbE patients.

3. Green tea for thalassemia's health

Green tea is prepared without fermentation from tea leaves and one of the most popular beverages in the world. It is composed of proteins, amino acids (e.g., 5-methylglutamine, glutamic acid, tryptophan, glycine, serine, aspartic acid, tyrosine, valine, leucine, threonine, arginine, and lysine), carbohydrates (e.g., cellulose, pectin, glucose, fructose, and sucrose), lipids (e.g., linoleic acid and α-linolenic acids), sterols (e.g., stigmasterol), vitamin B, vitamin C, vitamin E, caffeine, theophylline, chlorophyll, carotenoids, volatile compounds (e.g., aldehydes, alcohols, esters, lactones, and short-chain hydrocarbons), minerals, and essential elements. Importantly, green tea is rich in polyphenols, particularly flavonoids (0.5–1.5%) in forms of catechins (flavan-3-ols). Five main green tea catechins (GTC) are included, EGCG which is the main proportion (59% of total catechins), (−)-epigallocatechin (EGC), (−)-epicatechin-3-gallate (ECG), and (−)-epicatechin (EC) (**Figure 4**). In addition, green tea contains gallic acid, chlorogenic acid, caffeic acid, kaempferol, myricetin, and quercetin. During the fermentation process, flavonoids in green tea are oxidized into theaflavins and thearubigins, which are the main ingredients in black tea.

In health benefits, green tea plays many important roles in cells and systems in the body. Green tea has been considered a medicine and a healthful beverage since ancient times. Traditional Chinese medicine has recommended this plant for headaches, body aches and pains, digestion, depression, detoxification, as an energizer, and, in general, to prolong life. Caffeine acts mainly upon the central nervous system, stimulating wakefulness, facilitating ideas association, and decreasing the sensation of fatigue [73]. Green tea polyphenols present antioxidant, ROS and reactive nitrogen species (RNS) scavenging, and metal-chelating activities [72, 74, 75]. They may also function indirectly through (1) inhibition of redox-sensitive transcription factors; (2) inhibition of "prooxidant" enzymes including inducible nitric oxide synthase (iNOS), lipoxygenase (LOX), cyclooxygenase (COX), and xanthine oxidase (XO); and (3) induction of antioxidant enzymes including GST and SOD [76].

3.1 Neuronal cells

We have presented that GTE treatment at 0–100 μg/mL was not toxic to the neuroblastoma (SH SY5Y) cells (viability >90%). Nevertheless, the cell viability significantly decreased in iron-loaded condition, and the treatment of the cells with GTE (10–40 μg/mL) was found to improve the viability. GTE monotherapy (10–20 μM) was not effective to reduce LIP levels in SH SY5S cells, whereas combined treatment with GTE and CM1 iron chelator significantly reduced the LIP.

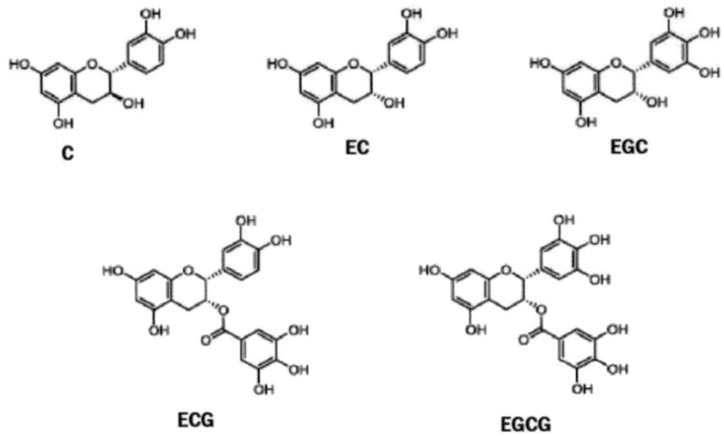

Figure 4.
Chemical structures of five catechins in green tea (modified from [72]). Abbreviations: C = catechin, EC = epicatechin, ECG = epicatechin-3-gallate, EGC = epigallocatechin, EGCG = epigallocatechin-3-gallate.

Moreover, GTE monotherapy (40 μM), as well as the combination of GTE and CM1 chelator, exhibited significant free radical scavenging activity in a concentration-dependent manner [77]. Consistently, Xu and colleagues have reported that the oral administration of EGCG (25 mg/kg/day, 7 days) regulated the iron-export protein ferroportin in the substantia nigra and reduced oxidative stress in Parkinson's disease mice [78].

3.2 Blood cells

Phenolic acids (e.g., chlorogenic acid, caffeic acid, and gallic acid) and flavonols (e.g., kaempferol, myricetin, and quercetin) are present in green tea. GTE and EGCG, which show iron-chelating and antioxidant properties, decrease labile iron (e.g., NTBI and LPI) levels and consequently deplete lipid peroxidation as well as oxidative stress in both iron-loaded rats and thalassemic mice [73, 74]. The compounds were effective in the inhibition of RBC hemolysis, resulting in prolonged RBC lifespan and decreased iron deposition and oxidative damage in liver [75]. Logically, antioxidative GTE interferes duodenal absorption of dietary iron and iron-chelating properties in vitro and in vivo. The preparation also shows the inhibitory effect on catecholamine secretion from isolated rabbit adrenal glands, possibly by blocking LTCC in the adrenomedullary glands. Active compounds in GTE are effective in the inhibition of red blood cell hemolysis; therefore, red blood cell lifespan can be expanded, and iron deposition in the liver can be decreased [79]. Green tea extract improves the abnormality of sickle red cells [80]. Using fluorochrome labeling and flow cytometry, we found feeding ferrocene diet-induced iron overload and oxidative stress, leading to a significant decrease of RBC survival half-time ($T_{1/2}$) in WT ($T_{1/2}$ = 23 days) and BKO thalassemic mice ($T_{1/2}$ = 13 days) when compared with feeding normal diet ($T_{1/2}$ = 30 days). Surprisingly, the RBC survival rate was approximately 15% increase in GTE-treated WT mice and 27% increase in GTE-treated BKO mice when compared with placebo-treated WT mice (Ounjaijean, S. unpublished data). Antioxidative GTE, particularly EGCG, would possibly scavenge ROS and recycle oxidized glutathione (GSSG) to GSH in RBC cytoplasm, leading to the inhibition of RBC hemolysis and prolonged RBC survival. Tea extracts can be used as a therapeutic agent in case of anemia resulting from red blood cell destruction and alleviate infection-induced inflammation or other inflammatory diseases [81, 82]. EGCG is presented to ameliorate inflammation via the nuclear factor erythroid-derived 2-like-2 (Nrf2 signaling pathway), leading to prevent osteoblasts [83]. On the other hand, excessive green tea consumption may cause iron-deficiency anemia [67].

3.3 Liver and pancreas cells

By using lactate dehydrogenase assay, Koonyosying and colleagues have found that GTE at 1–10 μM EGCG equivalent was not toxic to rat insulinoma (RINm-5F) cells, whereas GTE doses of 1–30 μM EGCG equivalent were not toxic to human hepatocellular carcinoma (Huh7) cells either, showing 20% inhibitory concentrations (IC20) of 10.6 and 17.4 μM EGCG equivalent, respectively [84]. Interestingly, GTE monotherapy (10 μM EGCG equivalent) revealed an almost twofold reduction of LIP in iron-loaded RINm-5F and Huh7 cells when compared to treatment without GTE, while GTE treatment (1 and 10 μM EGCG equivalent) together with 10 μM DFO showed a synergistic effect of the LIP mobilization. Similarly, the GTE treatments efficiently lowered ROS levels in these two cells in the same manner. Most importantly, the GTE treatments effectively restored the production of insulin from iron-loaded RINm-5F cells and hepcidin production from iron-loaded Huh7 cells, indicating relief of endocrine gland dysfunction from iron-induced oxidative tissue damage [84].

3.4 Hypercoagulability and thrombosis in thalassemia

Oral green tea catechins significantly inhibited arachidonic acid (AA)-induced platelet aggregation in rats [85]. Likewise, EGCG suppressed adenosine diphosphate (ADP)-induced platelet aggregation in a dose-dependent manner and reduced the ADP-induced phosphorylation of p38 mitogen-activated protein kinase and heat shock protein [86]. In addition, EGCG inhibited the ADP-stimulated release of platelet-derived growth factor-AB and soluble CD40 ligand [87]. Moreover, green tea catechins inhibited ATP release from dense granules in washed platelets and AA liberation stimulated by collagen in platelets [85]. Interestingly, GTC and EGCG prevented death due to pulmonary thrombosis, prolonged bleeding time in mice in vivo, and inhibited human platelet aggregation [88]. Nowadays, the life expectancy of TM patients has been improved because of regular blood transfusions and iron chelation therapy. However, patients with thalassemia still suffer from many complications from their chronic disease. Regular transfusion therapy leads to iron overload-related complications including growth retardation, hypoparathyroidism, diabetes and impaired glucose intolerance, osteoporosis, cardiomyopathy, liver fibrosis, and cirrhosis [89]. Heart failure and arrhythmia have been reported as the main cause of death in TM patients, whereas pulmonary hypertension and thrombosis are also the major cardiovascular complications in TI patients possibly due to pro-atherogenic biochemical factors (e.g., iron status and lipid profile) [90–94]. Hypercoagulable pulmonary microthromboembolism in Thai pediatric TE patients was previously investigated [95]. TI patients had thrombosis (9.4%), thrombocytosis (15%), mostly after splenectomy, and lower levels of anticoagulation inhibitors (e.g., protein S, protein C, and antithrombin III) (15%) [26]. Splenectomy also promotes portal vein thrombosis in TM patients [96]. Ineffective erythropoiesis, chronic anemia, iron overload, and polycythemia by erythrocytosis and thrombosis are coincidently occurring in patients with β-thalassemia. Signs of cerebrovascular accident (brain ischemia, hemorrhage, and infarct) and heart disease (congestive heart failure and atrial fibrillation) were described in patients with chronically hypercoagulable thromboembolic thalassemia, so anticoagulant and/or anti-platelet therapy is recommended [97].

According to a high incidence of coagulopathy affecting life expectancy, patients with thalassemia have been reported recently to understand contributing factors. Thrombosis related to the hypercoagulable state in thalassemia has been mostly reported. Factors contributing to the hypercoagulable state in patients have been identified [98]. Hypoxia and iron overload are the two major mechanisms of ROS overproduction that can cause oxidative tissue damage and complications [99]. The levels of plasma hemostatic and thrombotic markers including thrombin-antithrombin III complex, β2 thromboglobulin, C-reactive protein, tissue plasminogen activator antigen, protein C, protein S, antithrombin, prothrombin fragments, fibrinogen, and lipoprotein (a) were significantly higher in patients with splenectomized HbE/β-thalassemia than non-splenectomized ones, implying that splenectomy increases platelet hyperactivity, blood hypercoagulability, and risk of thrombosis [100, 101]. ROS-induced activation of vascular endothelial cells can cause vasculitis and thrombosis, showing increased levels of soluble adhesion molecules such as intercellular adhesion molecule-1 (ICAM-1), E-selectin (ELAM-1), vascular cell adhesion molecule-1 (VCAM-1), and von Willebrand factor (vWF) in thalassemia blood [102]. Procoagulant activity of circulating damaged RBC or RBC microvesicles may also contribute to thrombotic events in thalassemia hypercoagulability [103]. Carotid artery thrombus is usually associated with severe cardiovascular diseases (CVD), iron-deficiency anemia, and thrombocytosis. Thromboembolic complications are documented in patients with thalassemia, possibly due to the aggregability of abnormal RBC and high amounts of RBC membrane-derived microparticles [104]. The treatment of β-thalassemia/HbE patients with antioxidants can improve oxidative stress and hypercoagulable state [105]. Particularly, NTBI presenting in thalassemia plasma would be one of the risk factors in pulmonary thrombosis and hypertension in splenectomized NTDT patients [106]. DFO and DFP were effective in the amelioration of iron overload and oxidative stress in thalassemic mice, possibly in the prevention of pulmonary thrombosis [107].

Excessive iron and carbon monoxide liberated from heme oxygenase-1 catalyzed heme degradation also contribute to hypercoagulability [108]. Moreover, low arginine bioavailability and elevated arginase I activity in patients with β-thalassemia are possible causes of pulmonary hypertension leading to cardiopulmonary dysfunctions [109]. However, there are no difference in serum arginine between young patients with β-thalassemia and young control children [110]. Anemia (e.g., iron-deficiency anemia) can be linked to cerebral venous thrombosis as well [111]. Ex vivo Hb released from old RBC and in vivo Hb released from thalassemia RBC per se directly bind nitric oxide, whereas arginase will degrade available arginine during hemolysis [112]. Splenectomy, thrombocytosis, and only platelet MP are proposed to be residual hypercoagulable/thrombotic risks in TDT patients [23, 113]. Liver diseases such as liver inflammation and cirrhosis can involve in hypercoagulability, thrombosis, and reduced fibrinolysis [114, 115].

3.5 β-Thalassemic mice

Upanan and colleagues have demonstrated that hepatic hepcidin gene (Hamp1) mRNA levels in heterozygous β-globin knockout thalassemic mice (BKO, muβth-3/+) were significantly lower than that in wild-type mice (WT, muβ+/+) and significantly upregulated with iron loading. However, combined treatment of DFP (50 mg/kg) and GTE (50 mg EGCG equivalent) for 90 days was more effective in the upregulation of the Hamp1 mRNA levels in BKO thalassemic mice significantly. Similarly, monotherapy with the GTE effectively decreased serum levels of alanine aminotransferase in BKO thalassemic mice ($\Delta 11 + 9$ U/L), while the combined

GTE/DFP chelation showed greater effect (Δ1 + 9 U/L) ($P < 0.05$) when compared without GTE (Δ17 + 12 U/L), suggesting protection of oxidative liver damage. Likewise, GTE monotherapy and GTE plus DFP therapy was found to lower the levels of serum NTBI, spleen, and liver iron from iron-loaded BKO mice significantly when compared without GTE treatment [84, 116]. Currently, Al-Basher has shown that oral administration of GTE (100 mg/kg) for two more months lowered iron

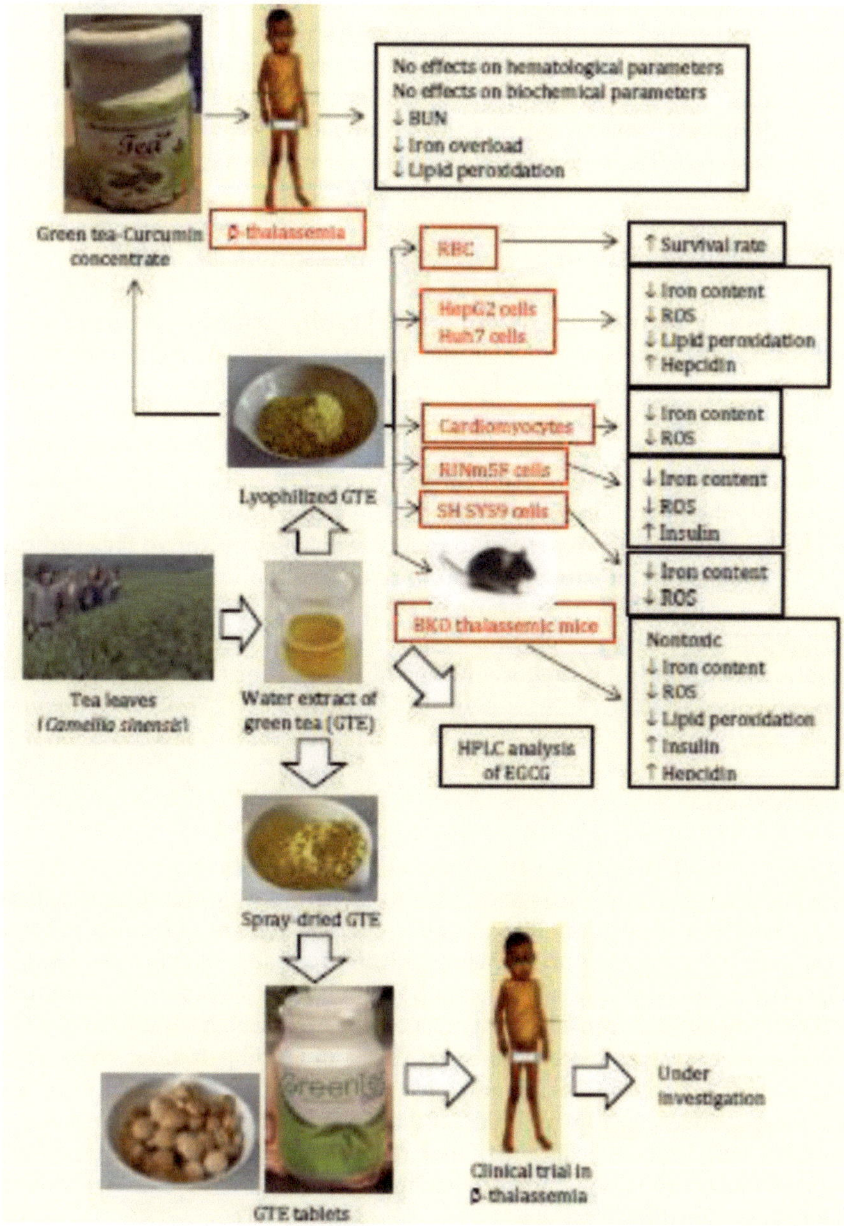

Figure 5.
Challenging with green tea for treatments of iron overload and oxidative: from cells to bedsides. Abbreviations/symbols: BKO = β-globin knockout, BUN = blood urea nitrogen, EGCG = epigallocatechin-3-gallate, GTE = green tea extract, HepG2 cells = human hepatocellular carcinoma cells, HPLC = high-performance liquid chromatography, Huh7 cells = human hepatocellular carcinoma cells, RBC = red blood cells, RINm5F cells = rat insulinoma cells, ROS = reactive oxygen species, SH SYS9 = human neuroblastoma cells, red alphabet = iron overload.

accumulation, improved antioxidant capacity, and restored the increase of hepcidin in the livers of iron-overloaded rats [117]. Recently, Koonyosying and colleagues have demonstrated that GTE decreased the amounts of iron in the livers ($P < 0.05$) and pancreas insignificantly from iron-loaded BKO mice; however, combination therapy of DFP and GTE was not efficient superior to the GTE monotherapy in the two cells [84]. Similarly, GTE treatment efficiently lowered the levels of lipid peroxidation products such as plasma TBARS and tissue MDA in liver and pancreatic tissues from BKO mice fed with ferrocene diet, and the combined treatment was not superior to the GTE monotherapy either [84]. Consistent with studies of the cells, GTE restored the production of hepatic hepcidin and pancreatic insulin in iron-loaded BKO mice, and the combined treatment was not more efficient over the GTE monotherapy [84]. The findings suggest protective effects of iron-induced oxidative hepatic and pancreatic damages by GTE, which the action would be mainly free radical scavenging property.

3.6 Patients with β-thalassemia

A recent study of controlled trial in British healthy volunteers has demonstrated that the interval between meal consumption and tea consumption did not affect plasma levels of hepcidin-25 [118]. Surprisingly, the consumption of GTE-curcumin drinks for 60 days tentatively decreased the levels of Hb, Hct, and RBC numbers in TDT patients [84]. Moreover, the drink with the GTE dose of 50 mg EGCG equivalent was found to lower the levels of NTBI and LPI. Taken together, green tea polyphenols and curcuminoids present in the drink could possibly interfere absorption of dietary iron and mobilize delivery of iron to the erythrons [65, 79, 119]. Taken all our studies, we summarize the applications of nutraceutical green tea extract for the amelioration of iron-overloaded cells, β-thalassemic mice, and patients with β-thalassemia (**Figure 5**) [79, 84, 106, 116, 119–128]. In our expectations, we hope the patients will have safer chelation therapy, a better quality of lives, and good health.

4. Conclusions

Patients with β-thalassemia suffer from ineffective erythropoiesis and chronic anemia and from secondary iron overload caused by multiple blood transfusions and increased iron absorption. Iron chelation therapy and antioxidant administration are supportive treatments to ameliorate iron overload and oxidative tissue damage. Green tea (*Camellia sinensis*) abundant with EGCG possesses diuretic, free radical scavenging, and iron-chelating properties. Accordingly, green tea products can decrease the levels of redox-active iron, ROS, and lipid peroxidation products in iron-overloaded cells, β-thalassemic mice, and patients. In addition, green tea can restore pancreatic insulin secretion and hepatic hepcidin production from hepatocytes with iron overload. Furthermore, the nutraceutical properties of green tea products have to be investigated intensively in patients with oxidative stress and neurodegenerative disorders.

Acknowledgements

We gratefully acknowledge Thailand Science Research and Innovation (Academic Section) (Grant number RGU6180007) and the Faculty of Medicine

Endowment Fund, Chiang Mai University, through Associate Professor Somdet Srichairatanakool, PhD., for providing funding.

Conflict of interest

The authors declare no conflict of interest.

Thanks

We also thank Dr. Narisara Paradee, Ph.D., for graphic and artwork and Mr. Touchwin Petiwathayakorn for supplying information on green tea.

Abbreviations

AA	arachidonic acid
ADP	adenosine 5′-phosphate
AE2	anion-exchange protein 2
ARE	antioxidant responsive element
ATP	adenosine-5′-triphosphate
BKO	beta-globin knockout
BUN	blood urea nitrogen
CAT	catalase
CH	chelator
COX	cyclooxygenase
DFO	desferrioxamine
DFP	deferiprone
DFX	deferasirox
DMT1	divalent metal ion transporter 1
EC	epicatechin
ECG	epicatechin-3-gallate
EGC	epigallocatechin
EGCG	epigallocatechin-3-gallate
EPO	erythropoietin
ERFE	erythroferrone
Fe	iron
Fe^{2+}	ferrous ion
Fe^{3+}	ferric ion
GI	gastrointestinal
GPx	glutathione peroxidase
GR	glutathione reductase
GSH	reduced glutathione
GSSG	oxidized glutathione
GST	glutathione-*S*-transferase
GTC	green tea catechins
GTE	green tea extract
Hamp1	hepatic hepcidin gene
Hb	hemoglobin
HbA	hemoglobin A
HbA_2	hemoglobin A_2

Hct	hematocrit
HbE	hemoglobin E
HbF	fetal hemoglobin
HbH	hemoglobin H
HepG2	human hepatocellular carcinoma cells
H_2O_2	hydrogen peroxide
HPLC	high-performance liquid chromatography
Huh7	human hepatocellular carcinoma cells
IC_{20}	20% inhibitory concentrations
iNOS	inducible nitric oxide synthase
IRE	iron regulatory element
IRP	iron regulatory protein
LIC	liver iron concentration
LIP	labile iron pools
LOX	lipoxygenase
LPI	labile iron pool
LTCC	L-type calcium channel
MDA	malondialdehyde
MP	microparticles
NAC	*N*-acetylcysteine
NFκB	nuclear factor-kappa B
Nrf2	nuclear factor erythroid 2
NTBI	non-transferrin-bound iron
Nramp2	natural resistance-associated macrophage protein 2
NTDT	non-transfusion-dependent β-thalassemia
$OH^{\bullet}$	hydroxyl radical
Prx2	peroxiredoxin 2
RBC	red blood cells
RE	reticuloendothelial
RINm5F	rat insulinoma cells
RNS	reactive nitrogen species
ROS	reactive oxygen species
SH SY5Y	neuroblastoma cells
SOD	superoxide dismutase
$T_{1/2}$	half-time
TBARS	thiobarbituric acid-reactive substances
TBI	transferrin-bound iron
TDT	transfusion-dependent β-thalassemia
Tf	transferrin
TfR1	transferrin receptor 1
TGF-β1	tumor growth factor-beta1
TI	β-thalassemia intermedia
TIBC	transferrin iron-binding capacity
TM	β-thalassemia major
TTCC	T-type calcium channel
TTCC	T-type calcium channel
XO	xanthine oxidase

Author details

Pimpisid Koonyosying[1], Suthat Fucharoen[2] and Somdet Srichairatanakool[1]*

1 Department of Biochemistry, Faculty of Medicine, Chiang Mai University, Chiang Mai, Thailand

2 Thalassemia Research Center, Institute of Molecular Biosciences, Mahidol University, Salaya Campus, Nakorn Pathom, Thailand

*Address all correspondence to: somdet.s@cmu.ac.th

References

[1] Taher A, Hershko C, Cappellini MD. Iron overload in thalassaemia intermedia: Reassessment of iron chelation strategies. British Journal of Haematology. 2009;**147**(5):634-640

[2] Kushner JP, Porter JP, Olivieri NF. Secondary iron overload. Hematology. American Society of Hematology. Education Program. 2001;**2001**(1):47-61

[3] Rund D, Rachmilewitz E. Beta-thalassemia. The New England Journal of Medicine. 2005;**353**(11):1135-1146

[4] Ricerca BM, Di Girolamo A, Rund D. Infections in thalassemia and hemoglobinopathies: Focus on therapy-related complications. Mediterranean Journal of Hematology and Infectious Diseases. 2009;**1**(1):e2009028

[5] Hershko C, Konijn AM, Link G. Iron chelators for thalassaemia. British Journal of Haematology. 1998;**101**(3):399-406

[6] Breuer W, Hershko C, Cabantchik ZI. The importance of non-transferrin bound iron in disorders of iron metabolism. Transfusion Science. 2000;**23**(3):185-192

[7] Coffey R, Knutson MD. The plasma membrane metal-ion transporter ZIP14 contributes to nontransferrin-bound iron uptake by human beta-cells. American Journal of Physiology. Cell Physiology. 2016;**312**(2):C169-CC75

[8] Garrick LM, Dolan KG, Romano MA, Garrick MD. Non-transferrin-bound iron uptake in Belgrade and normal rat erythroid cells. Journal of Cellular Physiology. 1999;**178**(3):349-358

[9] Ghio AJ, Nozik-Grayck E, Turi J, Jaspers I, Mercatante DR, Kole R, et al. Superoxide-dependent iron uptake: A new role for anion exchange protein 2. American Journal of Respiratory Cell and Molecular Biology. 2003;**29**(6):653-660

[10] Haldar S, Tripathi A, Qian J, Beserra A, Suda S, McElwee M, et al. Prion protein promotes kidney iron uptake via its ferrireductase activity. The Journal of Biological Chemistry. 2015;**290**(9):5512-5522

[11] Ji C, Kosman DJ. Molecular mechanisms of non-transferrin-bound and transferring-bound iron uptake in primary hippocampal neurons. Journal of Neurochemistry. 2015;**133**(5):668-683

[12] Lane DJ, Robinson SR, Czerwinska H, Bishop GM, Lawen A. Two routes of iron accumulation in astrocytes: Ascorbate-dependent ferrous iron uptake via the divalent metal transporter (DMT1) plus an independent route for ferric iron. The Biochemical Journal. 2010;**432**(1):123-132

[13] Liuzzi JP, Aydemir F, Nam H, Knutson MD, Cousins RJ. Zip14 (Slc39a14) mediates non-transferrin-bound iron uptake into cells. Proceedings of the National Academy of Sciences of the United States of America. 2006;**103**(37):13612-13617

[14] van Raaij SEG, Srai SKS, Swinkels DW, van Swelm RPL. Iron uptake by ZIP8 and ZIP14 in human proximal tubular epithelial cells. Biometals. 2019;**32**(2):211-226

[15] Esposito BP, Breuer W, Sirankapracha P, Pootrakul P, Hershko C, Cabantchik ZI. Labile plasma iron in iron overload: Redox activity and susceptibility to chelation. Blood. 2003;**102**(7):2670-2677

[16] Origa R, Galanello R, Ganz T, Giagu N, Maccioni L, Faa G, et al. Liver

iron concentrations and urinary hepcidin in beta-thalassemia. Haematologica. 2007;**92**(5):583-588

[17] Wang J, Pantopoulos K. Regulation of cellular iron metabolism. The Biochemical Journal. 2011;**434**(3): 365-381

[18] Abdalla MY, Fawzi M, Al-Maloul SR, El-Banna N, Tayyem RF, Ahmad IM. Increased oxidative stress and iron overload in Jordanian beta-thalassemic children. Hemoglobin. 2011;**35**(1):67-79

[19] Aphinives C, Kukongviriyapan U, Jetsrisuparb A, Kukongviriyapan V, Somparn N. Impaired endothelial function in pediatric hemoglobin E/beta-thalassemia patients with iron overload. The Southeast Asian Journal of Tropical Medicine and Public Health. 2015;**45**(6):1454-1463

[20] Hossain MF, Ismail M, Tanu AR, Shekhar HU. Respiratory burst enzymes, pro-oxidants and antioxidants status in Bangladeshi population with beta-thalassemia major. North American Journal of Medical Sciences. 2015;**7**(6):253-258

[21] Ozturk Z, Genc GE, Kupesiz A, Kurtoglu E, Gumuslu S. Thalassemia major patients using iron chelators showed a reduced plasma thioredoxin level and reduced thioredoxin reductase activity, despite elevated oxidative stress. Free Radical Research. 2015;**49**(3):309-316

[22] Wang WJ, Wu ZK, Zhang XH, Liu YM, Fang SP, Zhang C, et al. Effect of Yisui Shengxue granule on the oxidative damage of erythrocytes from patients with hemoglobin H disease. Chinese Journal of Integrative Medicine. 2012;**18**(9):670-675

[23] Agouti I, Cointe S, Robert S, Judicone C, Loundou A, Driss F, et al. Plateletandnoterythrocytemicroparticles are procoagulant in transfused thalassaemia major patients. British Journal of Haematology. 2015;**171**(4):615-624

[24] Amer J, Fibach E. Oxidative status of platelets in normal and thalassemic blood. Thrombosis and Haemostasis. 2004;**92**(5):1052-1059

[25] Atichartakarn V, Chuncharunee S, Archararit N, Udomsubpayakul U, Aryurachai K. Intravascular hemolysis, vascular endothelial cell activation and thrombophilia in splenectomized patients with hemoglobin E/beta-thalassemia disease. Acta Haematologica. 2014;**132**(1):100-107

[26] Bhattacharyya M, Kannan M, Chaudhry VP, Mahapatra M, Pati H, Saxena R. Hypercoagulable state in five thalassemia intermedia patients. Clinical and Applied Thrombosis/Hemostasis. 2007;**13**(4):422-427

[27] Okon E, Levij IS, Rachmilewitz EA. Splenectomy, iron overload and liver cirrhosis in beta-thalassemia major. Acta Haematologica. 1976;**56**(3):142-150

[28] Matsuno T, Mori M, Awai M. Distribution of ferritin and hemosiderin in the liver, spleen and bone marrow of normal, phlebotomized and iron overloaded rats. Acta Medica Okayama. 1985;**39**(5):347-360

[29] Legssyer R, Josse C, Piette J, Ward RJ, Crichton RR. Changes in function of iron-loaded alveolar macrophages after in vivo administration of desferrioxamine and/or chloroquine. Journal of Inorganic Biochemistry. 2003;**94**(1-2):36-42

[30] Matte A, De Falco L, Iolascon A, Mohandas N, An X, Siciliano A, et al. The interplay between peroxiredoxin-2 and nuclear factor-erythroid 2 is important in limiting oxidative

mediated dysfunction in beta-thalassemic erythropoiesis. Antioxidants & Redox Signaling. 2015;**23**(16):1284-1297

[31] Jensen PD. Evaluation of iron overload. British Journal of Haematology. 2004;**124**(6):697-711

[32] Deugnier Y, Turlin B, Ropert M, Cappellini MD, Porter JB, Giannone V, et al. Improvement in liver pathology of patients with beta-thalassemia treated with deferasirox for at least 3 years. Gastroenterology. [Randomized Controlled Trial Research Support, Non-U.S. Gov't]. 2011;**141**(4):1202-1211

[33] Chattipakorn N, Kumfu S, Fucharoen S, Chattipakorn S. Calcium channels and iron uptake into the heart. World Journal of Cardiology. 2011;**3**(7):215-218

[34] Deugnier Y, Turlin B. Pathology of hepatic iron overload. Seminars in Liver Disease. 2011;**31**(3):260-271

[35] Khamseekaew J, Kumfu S, Palee S, Wongjaikam S, Srichairatanakool S, Fucharoen S, et al. Effects of the iron chelator deferiprone and the T-type calcium channel blocker efonidipine on cardiac function and Ca(2+) regulation in iron-overloaded thalassemic mice. Cell Calcium. 2018;**72**:18-25

[36] Wolfe L, Olivieri N, Sallan D, Colan S, Rose V, Propper R, et al. Prevention of cardiac disease by subcutaneous deferoxamine in patients with thalassemia major. The New England Journal of Medicine. 1985;**312**(25):1600-1603

[37] Freeman AP, Giles RW, Berdoukas VA, Talley PA, Murray IP. Sustained normalization of cardiac function by chelation therapy in thalassaemia major. Clinical and Laboratory Haematology. 1989;**11**(4):299-307

[38] Brink B, Disler P, Lynch S, Jacobs P, Charlton R, Bothwell T. Patterns of iron storage in dietary iron overload and idiopathic hemochromatosis. The Journal of Laboratory and Clinical Medicine. 1976;**88**(5):725-731

[39] Soliman AT, elZalabany MM, Mazloum Y, Bedair SM, Ragab MS, Rogol AD, et al. Spontaneous and provoked growth hormone (GH) secretion and insulin-like growth factor I (IGF-I) concentration in patients with beta thalassaemia and delayed growth. Journal of Tropical Pediatrics. 1999;**45**(6):327-337

[40] Wood JC, Noetzl L, Hyderi A, Joukar M, Coates T, Mittelman S. Predicting pituitary iron and endocrine dysfunction. Annals of the New York Academy of Sciences. 2010;**1202**:123-128

[41] Nakavachara P, Viprakasit V. Adrenal insufficiency is prevalent in HbE/beta-thalassaemia paediatric patients irrespective of their clinical severity and transfusion requirement. Clinical Endocrinology. 2013;**79**(6):776-783

[42] Backe MB, Moen IW, Ellervik C, Hansen JB, Mandrup-Poulsen T. Iron regulation of pancreatic beta-cell functions and oxidative stress. Annual Review of Nutrition. 2016;**36**:241-273

[43] Jomova K, Valko M. Importance of iron chelation in free radical-induced oxidative stress and human disease. Current Pharmaceutical Design. 2011;**17**(31):3460-3473

[44] Andrews NC. Disorders of iron metabolism. The New England Journal of Medicine. 1999;**341**(26):1986-1995

[45] Cabantchik ZI, Breuer W, Zanninelli G, Cianciulli P. LPI-labile plasma iron in iron overload. Best Practice & Research. Clinical Haematology. 2005;**18**(2):277-287

[46] Cairo G, Recalcati S, Pietrangelo A, Minotti G. The iron regulatory proteins: Targets and modulators of free radical reactions and oxidative damage. Free Radical Biology & Medicine. 2002;**32**(12):1237-1243

[47] Yurkova I, Kisel M, Arnhold J, Shadyro O. Iron-mediated free-radical formation of signaling lipids in a model system. Chemistry and Physics of Lipids. 2005;**137**(1-2):29-37

[48] Schafer FQ, Qian SY, Buettner GR. Iron and free radical oxidations in cell membranes. Cellular and Molecular Biology (Noisy-le-Grand, France). 2000;**46**(3):657-662

[49] Youssry I, Mohsen NA, Shaker OG, El-Hennawy A, Fawzy R, Abu-Zeid NM, et al. Skin iron concentration: A simple, highly sensitive method for iron stores evaluation in thalassemia patients. Hemoglobin. 2007;**31**(3):357-365

[50] Mavrogeni SI, Markussis V, Kaklamanis L, Tsiapras D, Paraskevaidis I, Karavolias G, et al. A comparison of magnetic resonance imaging and cardiac biopsy in the evaluation of heart iron overload in patients with beta-thalassemia major. European Journal of Haematology. 2005;**75**(3):241-247

[51] Lee P, Mohammed N, Marshall L, Abeysinghe RD, Hider RC, Porter JB, et al. Intravenous infusion pharmacokinetics of desferrioxamine in thalassaemic patients. Drug Metabolism and Disposition. 1993;**21**(4):640-644

[52] Evans P, Kayyali R, Hider RC, Eccleston J, Porter JB. Mechanisms for the shuttling of plasma non-transferrin-bound iron (NTBI) onto deferoxamine by deferiprone. Translational Research. 2010;**156**(2):55-67

[53] Grady RW, Galanello R, Randolph RE, Kleinert DA, Dessi C, Giardina PJ. Toward optimizing the use of deferasirox: Potential benefits of combined use with deferoxamine. Haematologica. 2013;**98**(1):129-135

[54] Tanner MA, He T, Westwood MA, Firmin DN, Pennell DJ, Investigators TIFHT. Multi-center validation of the transferability of the magnetic resonance T2* technique for the quantification of tissue iron. Haematologica. 2006;**91**(10):1388-1391

[55] Porter JB, Faherty A, Stallibrass L, Brookman L, Hassan I, Howes C. A trial to investigate the relationship between DFO pharmacokinetics and metabolism and DFO-related toxicity. Annals of the New York Academy of Sciences. 1998;**850**:483-487

[56] Brittenham GM, Griffith PM, Nienhuis AW, McLaren CE, Young NS, Tucker EE, et al. Efficacy of deferoxamine in preventing complications of iron overload in patients with thalassemia major. The New England Journal of Medicine. 1994;**331**(9):567-573

[57] Farmaki K, Tzoumari I, Pappa C. Oral chelators in transfusion-dependent thalassemia major patients may prevent or reverse iron overload complications. Blood Cells, Molecules & Diseases. 2011;**47**(1):33-40

[58] Porter JB. Optimizing iron chelation strategies in beta-thalassaemia major. Blood Reviews. 2009;**23**(Suppl 1):S3-S7

[59] Vlachodimitropoulou Koumoutsea E, Garbowski M, Porter J. Synergistic intracellular iron chelation combinations: Mechanisms and conditions for optimizing iron mobilization. British Journal of Haematology. 2015;**170**(6):874-883

[60] Wapnick AA, Lynch SR, Krawitz P, Seftel HC, Charlton RW, Bothwell TH. Effects of iron overload on ascorbic acid metabolism. British Medical Journal. 1968;**3**(5620):704-707

[61] Chatterjea B, Maitra A, Banerjee DK, Basu AK. Status of ascorbic acid in iron deficiency anaemia and thalassaemia. Acta Haematologica. 1980;**64**(5):271-275

[62] Chapman RW, Hussain MA, Gorman A, Laulicht M, Politis D, Flynn DM, et al. Effect of ascorbic acid deficiency on serum ferritin concentration in patients with beta-thalassaemia major and iron overload. Journal of Clinical Pathology. 1982;**35**(5):487-491

[63] Dissayabutra T, Tosukhowong P, Seksan P. The benefits of vitamin C and vitamin E in children with beta-thalassemia with high oxidative stress. Journal of the Medical Association of Thailand. 2005;**88**(Suppl 4):S317-S321

[64] Fibach E, Rachmilewitz EA. The role of antioxidants and iron chelators in the treatment of oxidative stress in thalassemia. Annals of the New York Academy of Sciences. 2010;**1202**:10-16

[65] Kalpravidh RW, Siritanaratkul N, Insain P, Charoensakdi R, Panichkul N, Hatairaktham S, et al. Improvement in oxidative stress and antioxidant parameters in beta-thalassemia/ Hb E patients treated with curcuminoids. Clinical Biochemistry. 2009;**43**(4-5):424-429

[66] Unchern S, Laoharuangpanya N, Phumala N, Sipankapracha P, Pootrakul P, Fucharoen S, et al. The effects of vitamin E on platelet activity in beta-thalassaemia patients. British Journal of Haematology. 2003;**123**(4):738-744

[67] Fan FS. Iron deficiency anemia due to excessive green tea drinking. Clinical Case Reports. 2016;**4**(11):1053-1056

[68] Suzuki T, Pervin M, Goto S, Isemura M, Nakamura Y. Beneficial effects of tea and the green tea catechin epigallocatechin-3-gallate on obesity. Molecules. 2016;**21**(10):1305. DOI: 10.3390/molecules21101305

[69] Lou DQ, Nicolas G, Lesbordes JC, Viatte L, Grimber G, Szajnert MF, et al. Functional differences between hepcidin 1 and 2 in transgenic mice. Blood. 2004;**103**(7):2816-2821

[70] Zhang Y, Li H, Zhao Y, Gao Z. Dietary supplementation of baicalin and quercetin attenuates iron overload induced mouse liver injury. European Journal of Pharmacology. 2006;**535**(1-3):263-269

[71] Mullen W, Edwards CA, Crozier A. Absorption, excretion and metabolite profiling of methyl-, glucuronyl-, glucosyl- and sulpho-conjugates of quercetin in human plasma and urine after ingestion of onions. The British Journal of Nutrition. 2006;**96**(1):107-116

[72] McKay DL, Blumberg JB. The role of tea in human health: An update. Journal of the American College of Nutrition. 2002;**21**(1):1-13

[73] Varnam AH, Sutherland JP. Beverages: Technology, Chemistry and Microbiology. London: Chapman & Hall; 1994

[74] Kim J-H, Kang B-H, Jeong J-M. Antioxidant, antimutagenic and chemopreventive activities of a phyto-extract mixture derived from various vegetables, fruits, and oriental herbs. Food Science and Biotechnology. 2003;**12**(6):631-638

[75] Skrzydlewska E, Augustyniak A, Michalak K, Farbiszewski R. Green tea supplementation in rats of different ages mitigates ethanol-induced changes in brain antioxidant abilities. Alcohol. 2005;**37**(2):89-98

[76] Cabrera C, Artacho R, Gimenez R. Beneficial effects of green tea—A

review. Journal of the American College of Nutrition. 2006;**25**(2):79-99

[77] Chansiw N, Kulprachakarn K, Paradee N, Prommaban A, Srichairatanakool S. Neuroprotective effect of 1-(N-acetyl-6-aminohexyl)-3-hydroxy-2-methylpyridin-4-one iron chelator combined with green tea extract. Unpublished data

[78] Xu Q, Langley M, Kanthasamy AG, Reddy MB. Epigallocatechin gallate has a neurorescue effect in a mouse model of Parkinson disease. The Journal of Nutrition. 2017;**147**(10):1926-1931

[79] Saewong T, Ounjaijean S, Mundee Y, Pattanapanyasat K, Fucharoen S, Porter JB, et al. Effects of green tea on iron accumulation and oxidative stress in livers of iron-challenged thalassemic mice. Medicinal Chemistry. 2010;**6**(2):57-64

[80] Ohnishi ST, Ohnishi T, Ogunmola GB. Green tea extract and aged garlic extract inhibit anion transport and sickle cell dehydration in vitro. Blood Cells, Molecules & Diseases. 2001;**27**(1):148-157

[81] Karori SM, Ngure RM, Wachira FN, Wanyoko JK, Mwangi JN. Different types of tea products attenuate inflammation induced in *Trypanosoma brucei* infected mice. Parasitology International. 2008;**57**(3):325-333

[82] Ling JX, Wei F, Li N, Li JL, Chen LJ, Liu YY, et al. Amelioration of influenza virus-induced reactive oxygen species formation by epigallocatechin gallate derived from green tea. Acta Pharmacologica Sinica. 2012;**33**(12):1533-1541

[83] Liu S, Yang L, Mu S, Fu Q. Epigallocatechin-3-gallate ameliorates glucocorticoid-induced osteoporosis of rats in vivo and in vitro. Frontiers in Pharmacology. 2018;**9**:447

[84] Koonyosying P, Uthaipibull C, Fucharoen S, Koumoutsea EV, Porter JB, Srichairatanakool S. Decrement in cellular iron and reactive oxygen species, and improvement of insulin secretion in a pancreatic cell line using green tea extract. Pancreas. 2019;**48**(5):636-643

[85] Son DJ, Cho MR, Jin YR, Kim SY, Park YH, Lee SH, et al. Antiplatelet effect of green tea catechins: A possible mechanism through arachidonic acid pathway. Prostaglandins, Leukotrienes, and Essential Fatty Acids. 2004;**71**(1):25-31

[86] Hamann GL, Campbell JD, George CM. Warfarin-cranberry juice interaction. The Annals of Pharmacotherapy. 2011;**45**(3):e17

[87] Iida Y, Doi T, Matsushima-Nishiwaki R, Tokuda H, Ogura S, Kozawa O, et al. (−)-Epigallocatechin gallate selectively inhibits adenosine diphosphate-stimulated human platelet activation: Suppression of heat shock protein 27 phosphorylation via p38 mitogen-activated protein kinase. Molecular Medicine Reports. 2014;**10**(3):1383-1388

[88] Kang WS, Lim IH, Yuk DY, Chung KH, Park JB, Yoo HS, et al. Antithrombotic activities of green tea catechins and (−)-epigallocatechin gallate. Thrombosis Research. 1999;**96**(3):229-237

[89] Galanello R, Origa R. Beta-thalassemia. Orphanet Journal of Rare Diseases. 2010;**5**(1):11

[90] Cohen AR, Galanello R, Pennell DJ, Cunningham MJ, Vichinsky E. Thalassemia. Hematology. American Society of Hematology. Education Program. 2004;**2004**(1):14-34

[91] Lai ME, Vacquer S, Carta MP, Spiga A, Cocco P, Angius F, et al. Thalassemia intermedia is associated with a proatherogenic biochemical

phenotype. Blood Cells, Molecules & Diseases. 2011;**46**(4):294-299

[92] Eldor A, Rachmilewitz EA. The hypercoagulable state in thalassemia. Blood. 2002;**99**(1):36-43

[93] Taher AT, Otrock ZK, Uthman I, Cappellini MD. Thalassemia and hypercoagulability. Blood Reviews. 2008;**22**(5):283-292

[94] Wanachiwanawin W. Infections in E-beta thalassemia. Journal of Pediatric Hematology/Oncology. 2000;**22**(6):581-587

[95] Chuansumrit A, Hathirat P, Isarangkura P, Pintadit P, Mahaphan W. Thrombotic risk of children with thalassemia. Journal of the Medical Association of Thailand. 1993;**76** (Suppl 2):80-84

[96] Al-Hawsawi ZM, Haouimi AS, Hassan RA, Tarawah AM. Portal vein thrombosis after splenectomy for beta-thalassemia major. Saudi Medical Journal. 2004;**25**(2):225-228

[97] Karimi M, Khanlari M, Rachmilewitz EA. Cerebrovascular accident in beta-thalassemia major (beta-TM) and beta-thalassemia intermedia (beta-TI). American Journal of Hematology. 2008;**83**(1):77-79

[98] Cappellini MD, Musallam KM, Marcon A, Taher AT. Coagulopathy in beta-thalassemia: Current understanding and future perspectives. Mediterranean Journal of Hematology and Infectious Diseases. 2009;**1**(1):e2009029

[99] Tyan PI, Radwan AH, Eid A, Haddad AG, Wehbe D, Taher AT. Novel approach to reactive oxygen species in nontransfusion-dependent thalassemia. BioMed Research International. 2014;**2014**:8

[100] Angchaisuksiri P, Atichartakarn V, Aryurachai K, Archararit N, Chuncharunee S, Tiraganjana A, et al. Hemostatic and thrombotic markers in patients with hemoglobin E/beta-thalassemia disease. American Journal of Hematology. 2007;**82**(11):1001-1004

[101] Atichartakarn V, Angchaisuksiri P, Aryurachai K, Chuncharunee S, Thakkinstian A. In vivo platelet activation and hyperaggregation in hemoglobin E/beta-thalassemia: A consequence of splenectomy. International Journal of Hematology. 2003;**77**(3):299-303

[102] Butthep P, Bunyaratvej A, Funahara Y, Kitaguchi H, Fucharoen S, Sato S, et al. Possible evidence of endothelial cell activation and disturbance in thalassemia: An in vitro study. The Southeast Asian Journal of Tropical Medicine and Public Health. 1997;**28**(Suppl 3):141A-148A

[103] Cappellini MD, Grespi E, Cassinerio E, Bignamini D, Fiorelli G. Coagulation and splenectomy: An overview. Annals of the New York Academy of Sciences. 2005;**1054**:317-324

[104] Pattanapanyasat K, Gonwong S, Chaichompoo P, Noulsri E, Lerdwana S, Sukapirom K, et al. Activated platelet-derived microparticles in thalassaemia. British Journal of Haematology. 2007;**136**(3):462-471

[105] Yanpanitch O-U, Hatairaktham S, CharoensakdiR,PanichkulN,FucharoenS, Srichairatanakool S, et al. Treatment of beta-thalassemia/hemoglobin E with antioxidant cocktails results in decreased oxidative stress, increased hemoglobin concentration, and improvement of the hypercoagulable state. Oxidative Medicine and Cellular Longevity. 2015;**2015**:537954

[106] Inthawong K, Charoenkwan P, Silvilairat S, Tantiworawit A, Phrommintikul A, Choeyprasert W, et al. Pulmonary hypertension

in non-transfusion-dependent thalassemia: Correlation with clinical parameters, liver iron concentration, and non-transferrin-bound iron. Hematology. 2015;**20**(10):610-617

[107] Yatmark P, Morales NP, Chaisri U, Wichaiyo S, Hemstapat W, Srichairatanakool S, et al. Effects of iron chelators on pulmonary iron overload and oxidative stress in beta-thalassemic mice. Pharmacology. 2015;**96**(3-4):192-199

[108] Nielsen VG, Pretorius E. Iron and carbon monoxide enhance coagulation and attenuate fibrinolysis by different mechanisms. Blood Coagulation & Fibrinolysis. 2014;**25**(7):695-702

[109] Morris CR, Kim HY, Klings ES, Wood J, Porter JB, Trachtenberg F, et al. Dysregulated arginine metabolism and cardiopulmonary dysfunction in patients with thalassaemia. British Journal of Haematology. 2015;**169**(6):887-898

[110] Abdulrazzaq YM, Ibrahim A, Al-Khayat AI, Dawson K. Beta-thalassemia major and its effect on amino acid metabolism and growth in patients in the United Arab Emirates. Clinica Chimica Acta. 2005;**352**(1-2):183-190

[111] Stolz E, Valdueza JM, Grebe M, Schlachetzki F, Schmitt E, Madlener K, et al. Anemia as a risk factor for cerebral venous thrombosis? An old hypothesis revisited. Results of a prospective study. Journal of Neurology. 2007;**254**(6):729-734

[112] El-Hady SB, Farahat MH, Atfy M, Elhady MA. Nitric oxide metabolites and arginase I levels in beta-thalassemic patients: An Egyptian study. Annals of Hematology. 2012;**91**(8):1193-1200

[113] Musallam KM, Taher AT, Karimi M, Rachmilewitz EA. Cerebral infarction in beta-thalassemia intermedia: Breaking the silence. Thrombosis Research. 2012;**130**(5):695-702

[114] Gonzalez-Reimers E, Quintero-Platt G, Martin-Gonzalez C, Perez-Hernandez O, Romero-Acevedo L, Santolaria-Fernandez F. Thrombin activation and liver inflammation in advanced hepatitis C virus infection. World Journal of Gastroenterology. 2016;**22**(18):4427-4437

[115] Kell DB, Pretorius E. The simultaneous occurrence of both hypercoagulability and hypofibrinolysis in blood and serum during systemic inflammation, and the roles of iron and fibrin(ogen). Integrative Biology (Cambridge). 2015;**7**(1):24-52

[116] Upanan S, Pangjit K, Uthaipibull C, Fucharoen S, McKie AT, Srichairatanakool S. Combined treatment of 3-hydroxypyridine-4-one derivatives and green tea extract to induce hepcidin expression in iron-overloaded β-thalassemic mice. Asian Pacific Journal of Tropical Biomedicine. 2015;**5**(12):1010-1017

[117] Al-Basher GI. Green tea activity and iron overload induced molecular fibrogenesis of rat liver. Saudi Journal of Biological Sciences. 2019;**26**(3):531-540

[118] Ahmad Fuzi SF, Koller D, Bruggraber S, Pereira DI, Dainty JR, Mushtaq S. A 1-h time interval between a meal containing iron and consumption of tea attenuates the inhibitory effects on iron absorption: A controlled trial in a cohort of healthy UK women using a stable iron isotope. The American Journal of Clinical Nutrition. 2017;**106**(6):1413-1421

[119] Koonyosying P, Kongkarnka S, Uthaipibull C, Svasti S, Fucharoen S, Srichairatanakool S. Green tea extract modulates oxidative tissue injury in beta-thalassemic mice by chelation of redox iron and inhibition of

lipid peroxidation. Biomedicine & Pharmacotherapy. 2018;**108**:1694-1702

[120] Koonyosying P, Tantiworawit A, Hantrakool S, Utama-Ang N, Cresswell M, Fucharoen S, et al. Consumption of a green tea extract-curcumin drink decreases blood urea nitrogen and redox iron in beta-thalassemia patients. Food & Function. 2020;**11**(1):932-943

[121] Chansiw N, Pangjit K, Phisalaphong C, Porter JB, Evans P, Fucharoen S, et al. Effect of a novel oral active iron chelator: 1-(N-acetyl-6-aminohexyl)-3-hydroxy-2-methylpyridin-4-one (CM1) in iron-overloaded and non-overloaded mice. Asian Pacific Journal of Tropical Medicine. 2014;**7S1**:S155-S161

[122] Incharoen T, Thephinlap C, Srichairatanakool S, Chattipakorn S, Winichagoon P, Fucharoen S, et al. Heart rate variability in beta-thalassemic mice. International Journal of Cardiology. 2007;**121**(2):203-204

[123] Ounjaijean S, Thephinlap C, Khansuwan U, Phisalapong C, Fucharoen S, Porter JB, et al. Effect of green tea on iron status and oxidative stress in iron-loaded rats. Medicinal Chemistry. 2008;**4**(4):365-370

[124] Srichairatanakool S, Ounjaijean S, Thephinlap C, Khansuwan U, Phisalpong C, Fucharoen S. Iron-chelating and free-radical scavenging activities of microwave-processed green tea in iron overload. Hemoglobin. 2006;**30**(2):311-327

[125] Srichairatanakool S, Thephinlap C, Phisalaphong C, Porter JB, Fucharoen S. Curcumin contributes to in vitro removal of non-transferrin bound iron by deferiprone and desferrioxamine in thalassemic plasma. Medicinal Chemistry. 2007;**3**(5):469-474

[126] Thephinlap C, Ounjaijean S, Khansuwan U, Fucharoen S, Porter JB, Srichairatanakool S. Epigallocatechin-3-gallate and epicatechin-3-gallate from green tea decrease plasma non-transferrin bound iron and erythrocyte oxidative stress. Medicinal Chemistry. 2007;**3**(3):289-296

[127] Thephinlap C, Phisalaphong C, Lailerd N, Chattipakorn N, Winichagoon P, Vadolas J, et al. Reversal of cardiac iron loading and dysfunction in thalassemic mice by curcuminoids. Medicinal Chemistry. 2011;7(1):62-69

[128] Upanan S, McKie AT, Latunde-Dada GO, Roytrakul S, Uthaipibull C, Pothacharoen P, et al. Hepcidin suppression in beta-thalassemia is associated with the down-regulation of atonal homolog 8. International Journal of Hematology. 2017;**106**(2):196-205

Section 3

Pathophysiology of Beta Thalassemia

Chapter 5

Model Human β Thalassemic Erythrocytes: Effect of Unpaired Purified α-Hemoglobin Chains on Normal Erythrocytes

Mark D. Scott

Abstract

β thalassemias arise from genetic defects that interfere with the synthesis of the β hemoglobin chain and the subsequent production of the normal $\alpha_2\beta_2$ hemoglobin tetramer. As a consequence of this decreased β-chain synthesis, unpaired α-hemoglobin chains are found within the red blood cell (RBC). The unstable α-chains are associated with a number of cellular defects, including: membrane-bound globin; membrane thiol oxidation; altered cytoskeletal proteins; decreased cellular and membrane deformability; and increased susceptibility to both endogenous and exogenous oxidants. Surprisingly, while significant injury to human thalassemic RBC arise from the unpaired α-chains, the underlying intra-RBC mechanisms are not easily studied in patient samples or in mouse models. To better study the *fate of excess α-chains* in human RBC, the model β Thalassemic cell was developed. Model human β thalassemic RBC is made by entrapping purified human α-chains within normal RBC via osmotic lysis and resealing. This human model allows for the systematic examination of the mechanisms underlying the α-chain mediated damage in the β thalassemic RBC. Studies utilizing the model β thalassemic RBC have demonstrated that the α-chains give rise to an iron and glutathione-dependent, self-amplifying and self-propagating oxidative reaction.

Keywords: β thalassemia, α-hemoglobin chains, iron, red blood cell, erythrocyte, oxidation, free radicals, glutathione, deformability

1. Introduction

The thalassemias are a major cause of morbidity and mortality throughout much of the world [1–9]. Thalassemias are characterized by the disruption of the synthesis of normal adult hemoglobin (HbA; an $\alpha_2\beta_2$ tetramer; **Figure 1**) consequent to a diverse array of genetic mutations/deletions to either the β or α-hemoglobin chain genes (Chromosomes 11 and 16, respectively). As a consequence of reduced/absent production of β-chains, β thalassemia is characterized by the presence of highly unstable monomeric α-chains as these chains cannot self-associate and indeed require a chaperone protein to prevent precipitation [10]. In contrast, α thalassemia is characterized by the presence of relatively stable tetrameric β chains. Interestingly, as schematically shown in **Figure 1**, unlike most genes, there are four copies of the α-globin genes;

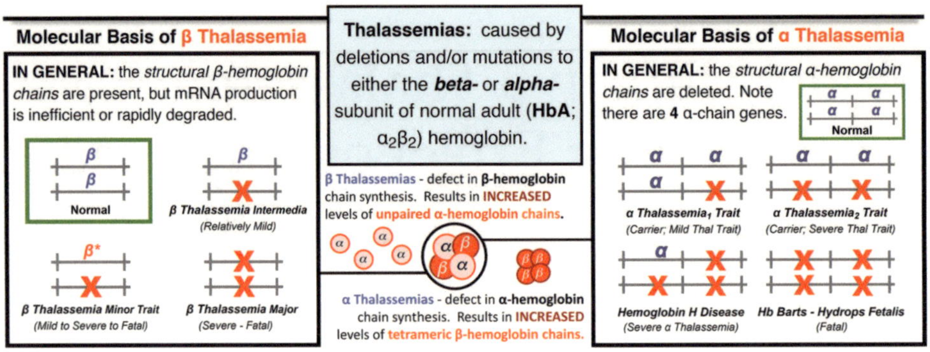

Figure 1.
Molecular basis and clinical diagnosis of the α and β thalassemias [1–9]. β denotes abnormal β hemoglobin gene such as HbS or HbE.*

this is in contrast to the expected two copies of the β-globin genes. The evolutionary duplication of the human α-chain genes may have been favored consequent to the inherent instability of monomeric α-chains. Indeed, the instability of the α-chains is the key factor underlying the pathophysiology of the β thalassemic red blood cell (RBC). Moreover, the pathophysiology of β thalassemia can be further complicated by the geographical prevalence, and high frequency, of a number of mutated β hemoglobin genes (e.g., sickle hemoglobin, hemoglobin E and hemoglobin C). If a mutated β-chain is the only functional β-chain present, the resultant disease will be more severe than that observed in β thalassemia Intermedia (a single normal β-globin gene). Loss of both β-chain genes gives rise to severe β Thalassemia Major which is fatal in the absence of transfusion therapy. The α thalassemias are characterized by a broader range of disease states due to the presence of 4 α genes. The loss of expression from a single gene (α $Thalassemia_1$ Trait) is often asymptomatic and undiagnosed; though the individual is a carrier for α Thalassemia and, in high frequency geographic areas may be at elevated risk for symptomatic disease transmission to an offspring. Deletion of two or three α-genes results in severe disease as a single active α-gene cannot, due to the instability of the chain, produce sufficient mature α-chains to form sufficient HbA. Loss of all four α-genes is fatal (resulting in Hydrops fetalis) due to the crucial role that α-chains play in embryonic and fetal hemoglobin. In contrast to β thalassemia, stable mutated α-chains are rare so typically these do not pose a significant complication in the pathophysiology of α thalassemia.

In this chapter we will further explore the pathophysiology of the β thalassemic RBC. Surprisingly, while significant injury to the thalassemic erythrocyte arises from the excess α-chains, the underlying mechanisms by which these chains damage and subsequently destroy the thalassemic RBC in the bone marrow and peripheral blood have not been clearly delineated. Our lack of understanding of the mechanisms of α-chain mediated damage is due, in part, to three major factors: (1) studies of RBC from β thalassemic individuals are difficult to do since these cells, upon collection, already exhibit significant injury and represent a survivorship bias since up to 80% of erythroid precursors are destroyed within the bone; (2) β thalassemic patients are typically transfused to both correct the severe anemia accompanying the disease and to prevent endogenous erythropoiesis of defective RBC; and (3) the lack of a good experimental model by which the pathophysiology of excess globin chains on human RBC can be examined.

While little can be done to change the first two problems, researchers have attempted to tackle the third issue using murine models of thalassemia [11–17]. Original murine studies examining the knockout of the murine β-chains were not productive as the murine α-chains behave significantly different from their human counterpart. To overcome this problem, human α-chain genes were inserted into the mouse genome in place of the murine genes. Again, these studies failed to give rise to as severe a phenotype as is seen in the human disease. Subsequent studies utilized additional mutations to produce symptomatic disease in the murine context—albeit with still substantial differences from the pathophysiology seen in the human β thalassemic RBC. Hence, an alternative approach for studying the pathophysiology of unpaired α-chains on the human RBC was needed.

2. Model human β thalassemic RBC

To this end, our laboratory developed an *in vitro* model of the HUMAN β thalassemic erythrocyte [18–27]. In this model, purified human α-chains are entrapped within normal human RBC (or, if desired, mouse RBC) by osmotic lysis and resealing (**Figure 2**) [18–34]. As previously shown, osmotic lysis and resealing results in RBC exhibiting normal hemoglobin concentration and volume (**Table 1**) as well as normal ATP concentration, oxidant sensitivity, morphology and

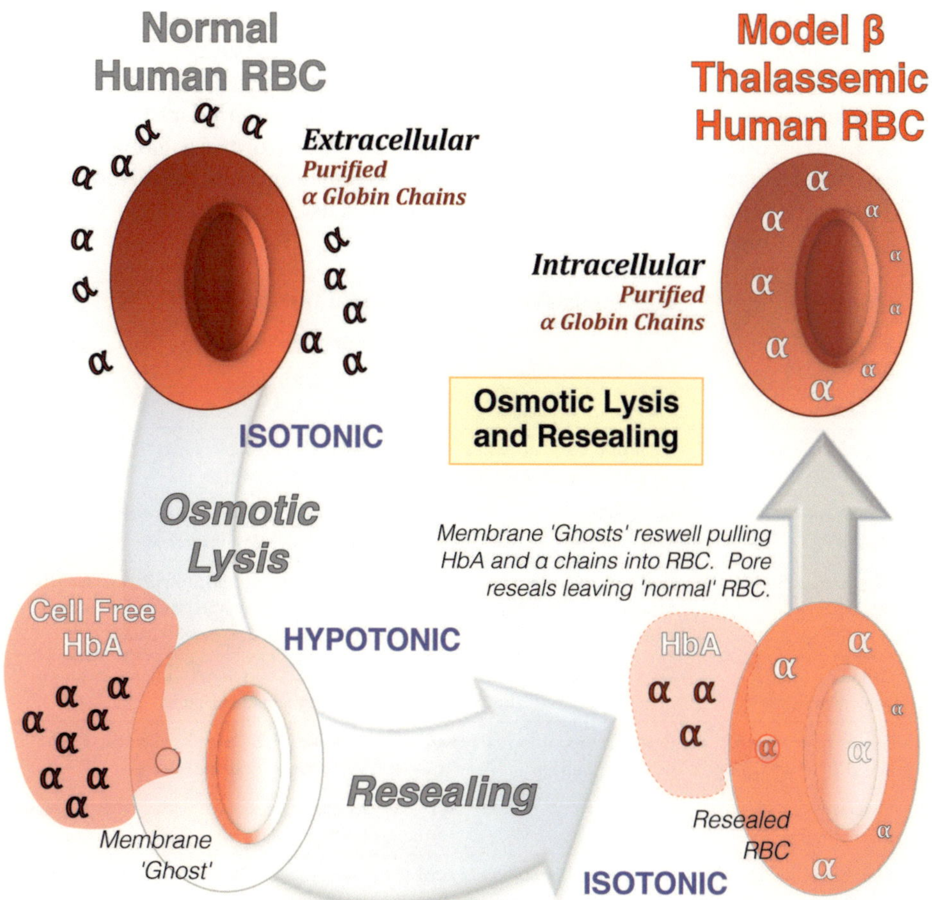

Figure 2.
Generation of model β thalassemic RBC from normal human donor cells via osmotic lysis and resealing [18–34]. Osmotically lysed and resealed RBC have normal morphology and metabolism and exhibit normal in vivo *survival.*

Parameter	N	Normal	Resealed*	Model β thal*	Model α thal*,**
Mean cell volume (μm^3)	7	88.9 ± 1.5	85.8 ± 4.5	78.6 ± 0.8	76.0 ± 4.0
Mean cell hemoglobin (pg)	7	30.5 ± 0.8	28.5 ± 2.7	23.4 ± 0.6	26.9 ± 2.1
Mean cell Hb conc. (g/dl)	7	34.2 ± 0.7	33.2 ± 1.7	29.6 ± 0.6	35.5 ± 1.3
Red cell distribution width (RDW)	7	12.9 ± 0.2	17.5 ± 4.5	29.2 ± 0.5	21.3 ± 3.8

**Immediately post resealing and washing 3×.*
***Made via the entrapment of purified human β hemoglobin chains.*

Table 1.
Cellular characteristics of model β and α thalassemic RBC [18–27].

deformability while allowing for the efficient entrapment of exogenous compounds [18–34]. Indeed, studies with resealed human RBC demonstrate that this methodology can be used to correct enzyme deficiencies, enhance antioxidant levels, and be used *in vitro* to study malarial growth and maturation. Moreover, murine studies demonstrated that osmotically resealed murine RBC exhibited normal *in vivo* survival. To manufacture the *model β thalassemic* RBC from normal human donor cells, purified, heme-containing, α-hemoglobin chains were prepared by dissociation of CO-treated HbA in the presence of parahydroxymercuribenzoate, followed by ion exchange chromatography, to isolate the purified CO-α-chains as previously described [1, 18, 20–22, 35, 36]. Analysis of the purified α-chains by mass spectroscopy demonstrated the expected mass values for the α-globin chain. The purified α-chains can be stored at −80°C as carbon monoxide stabilized chains (CO-α-chains) and then thawed immediately prior to use.

Characteristic	β thalassemic RBC	Model β thalassemic RBC
Microcytic RBC (MCV <80 fl)	+	+ (progressive)
K+ Loss	+	+
Unpaired α-chains	1–3% of total hemoglobin in peripheral blood reticulocytes	3–4% of total hemoglobin
Membrane Bound Globin	Increased	Increased; correlated with α-chain autoxidation & heme release.
Membrane proteins/ thiols	Loss of spectrin and ankyrin. Oxidation of membrane thiol (-SH) groups.	Loss of spectrin and ankyrin correlated with membrane thiol (-SH) oxidation, α-chain autoxidation, and heme release.
Cellular deformability	Decreased cellular and membrane deformability	Decreased; correlated with iron/heme deposition in membrane.
Intracellular oxidant stress	Evidence supporting increased oxidative damage	Increased H_2O_2; correlated with α-chain autoxidation & heme release.
Oxidant susceptibility	Increased	Increased; correlated with membrane bound iron/heme.
Membrane bound iron/heme	Increased membrane associated hemoglobin & Heinz body formation	Increased membrane heme; correlated with α-chain autoxidation.
Short in vivo survival	+	+ (*murine model β Thal RBC*)

Table 2.
Comparison of the pathologic characteristics of β thalassemic and model β thalassemic erythrocytes [18–27].

Entrapment of the purified α-chains within normal erythrocytes is done by osmotic lysis and resealing as previously described [18–34]. Briefly, washed, packed erythrocytes (80–85% hematocrit) are mixed with the purified CO-α-chains (10 mg/ml packed red cells) and then placed as a thin film within 11.5 mm diameter dialysis tubing (MW cutoff of 3500). The samples are dialyzed against a hypotonic lysis buffer (5 mM potassium phosphate buffer and 2 mM EDTA; pH 7.4) at 4°C for 60 min. The dialysis tubing is then transferred to an isotonic resealing buffer (5 mM potassium phosphate, 160 mM NaCl, and 5 mM glucose; pH 7.4) with gentle agitation for 30 min at 37°C. Following resealing, cells are washed with saline until the supernatant is clear. Using this procedure, approximately 70–80% of the initial packed erythrocyte volume is recovered. Radiolabeled α-chains can be utilized to quantitate the intracellular entrapment [18, 20].

To determine whether the model β thalassemic erythrocytes exhibit the cellular abnormalities characteristic of true β thalassemic cells, a number of cellular parameters have been examined. The results of these studies demonstrate that the α-chain loaded erythrocytes exhibit structural and functional changes very similar to those seen in β thalassemic erythrocytes (**Table 2**). Consequently, this model allowed for the systematic examination of the mechanisms underlying the α-chain mediated damage within the β thalassemic RBC and to directly determine the ontogeny of the pathologic events underlying the RBC injury and to experimentally test potential therapeutic approaches.

3. Iron-glutathione driven progeria of the thalassemic RBC

Containing approximately 20 mM iron, the RBC is the most ferruginous somatic cell in mammals. Under normal conditions, most of this iron is complexed within hemoglobin (as heme) with virtually none present as free metal (i.e., non-heme). This near perfect compartmentalization of iron may, however, break down in certain pathologic states such as β thalassemia and sickle cell disease resulting in the autoxidation of hemoglobin (i.e., formation of methemoglobin and hemichromes). Of physiologic importance, the monomeric α-chains spontaneously autoxidize to

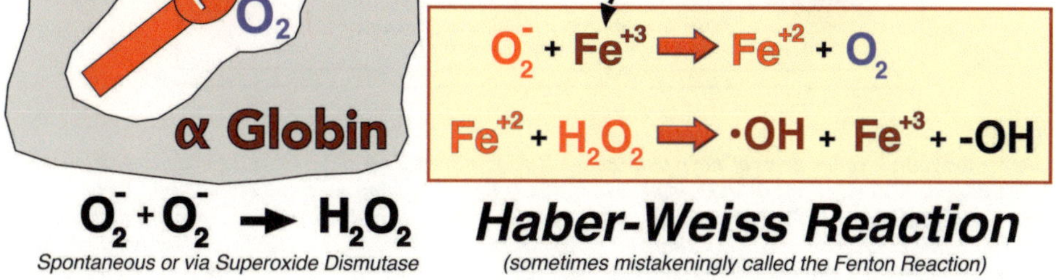

Figure 3.
Free radical basis of α-hemoglobin autoxidation and free radical injury. Consequent to the formation of methemoglobin, the non-covalently bound heme is 8-times more likely to escape the globin chain. Release of the heme initiates iron-dependent free radical reactions. References: [18–27].

methemoglobin, simultaneously generating superoxide (O_2^-), at a rate 8-times that of normal hemoglobin (**Figure 3**) [18, 20, 22–27, 37–39]. Moreover, consequent to the formation of methemoglobin, the non-covalently bound heme is more likely to escape the heme pocket of the globin chain giving rise to elevated levels of free, redox-active, intraerythrocytic iron. The O_2^- produced via the autoxidation of hemoglobin can reduce ferric (Fe^{+3}) to ferrous (Fe^{+2}) iron or form hydrogen peroxide (H_2O_2; either spontaneously or enzymatically via superoxide dismutase). Importantly, the iron, O_2^-, and H_2O_2 can, via the Haber-Weiss Reaction, give rise to the formation of the 'dreaded' hydroxyl radical (•OH) which rapidly reacts with virtually all biological constituents converting pristine materials into biological garbage (**Figure 3**). However, despite the general concept that free iron and the formation of free radicals are bad, the actual iron-dependent pathophysiology of the β thalassemic RBC has been poorly understood.

Mechanistically, studies using the model β thalassemic RBC have demonstrated that the initial autoxidation of the unpaired α-chains initiates an iron and reduced glutathione (GSH) dependent, self-amplifying and self-propagating reaction with the subsequent release of even more heme and, eventually, free iron. Schematically, this self-amplifying, self-propagating injury pathway is shown in **Figure 4**. As noted, the reaction process is initiated by the autoxidation of the unpaired α-chains which gives rise to the release of free heme and the generation of O_2^-. Interestingly, at this

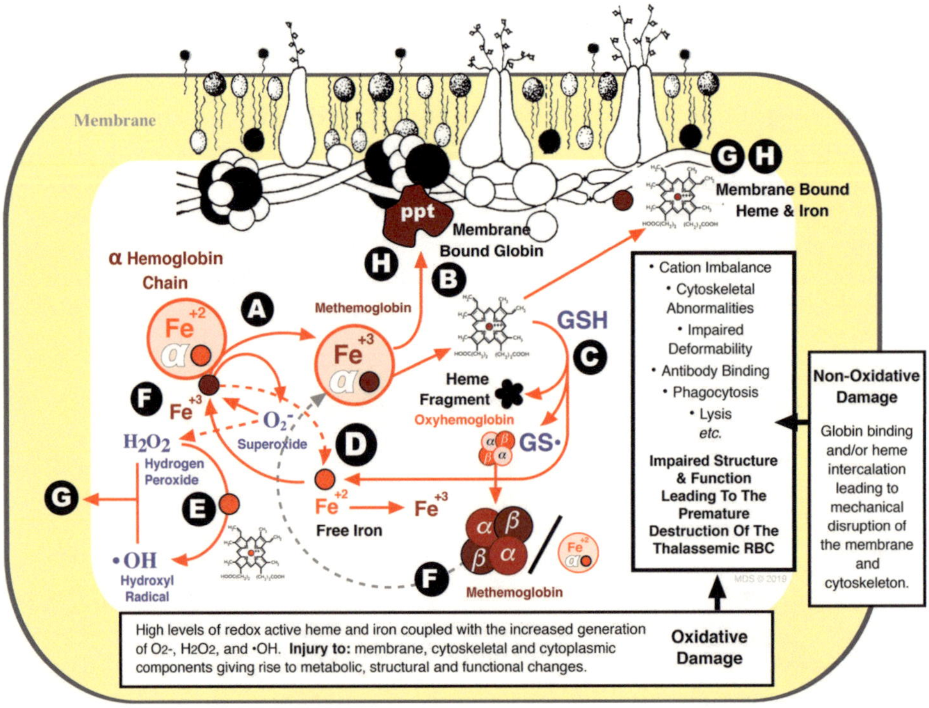

Figure 4.

Damage to multiple components of the β thalassemic RBC is mediated by an Fe-GSH dependent mechanism. As thalassemic RBC circulate, α-hemoglobin chains autoxidize (A) giving rise to superoxide (O_2^-) and methemoglobin [MetHb]. The heme moiety of the α metHb chains are released yielding free heme and globin (B). Free heme reacts with reduced glutathione [GSH; reaction (C)] resulting in cleavage of the heme group and the formation of a glutathione radical (GS•) and the release of free Fe^{+2} (D). The free iron (E) reacts with hemoglobin derived reactive oxygen species (ROS: O_2^- and H_2O_2) to generate •OH – A highly reactive radical capable of damaging all cellular components including cellular metabolism and cation/anion balance. The ferric iron (Fe^{+3}), in the presence of additional GSH or O_2^- regenerates Fe^{+2} which then oxidizes additional hemoglobin (F). Reactions (G) and (H) represent subsequent oxidative and non-oxidative injury to the cell. Oxidative pathway generated from references: [18–27, 40].

point, a key component of this pathway is GSH; an 'anti-oxidant' present at high intracellular (~2.3 mM) concentrations within the RBC [41, 42]. GSH readily reacts with free heme resulting in the cleavage of the heme ring, the release of free iron, and the formation of a thiol radical (GS•). This reaction leads to the rapid amplification of the oxidative damage to the RBC [18, 20, 22–27]. .The importance of the released iron and GSH was documented experimentally. As shown in **Figure 5A**, addition of Fe^{+3} to hemolysates from normal RBC results in the rapid oxidation of oxyhemoglobin in an iron-dose dependent manner. The oxidation of hemoglobin can be inhibited by the inclusion of an iron chelator (shown is deferoxamine; DFO) or by chemical depletion of GSH (not shown) [23, 27]. Moreover, in the intact model β thalassemic RBC, chemical depletion of GSH inhibited iron-driven hemoglobin oxidation (**Figure 5B**) [23, 27]. In contrast, as shown in **Figure 5C**, increasing the amount of intracellular GSH (via osmotic lysis and resealing; see **Figure 2**) in the model β thalassemic RBC significantly exacerbated injury to the cell. This enhanced injury is readily seen by the significantly reduced deformability (i.e., increased mean cell transit time) of the GSH-loaded model β thalassemic cells relative to the control model β thalassemic RBC. Importantly, as shown, GSH supplementation of normal RBC in the absence of iron had no detrimental effects on cellular deformability.

The enhanced oxidative stress, and consumption of GSH, was further noted by the time dependent decrease in GSH noted in the model β thalassemic RBC (**Table 3**) [27]. Moreover, a decrease in the NADPH/NADPtotal ratio was noted. NADPH is utilized to regenerate reduced GSH from oxidized (GSSG) glutathione via glutathione reductase. This decrease in the $NADPH/NADP_{total}$ ratio is likely reflective of both the high GSH-GSSG-GSH cycling but also of metabolic abnormalities arising consequent to iron and free radical mediated inhibition of normal glucose metabolism (**Figure 4**). Also of physiological importance, was the finding that the model β thalassemic RBC exhibited significantly ($p < 0.001$) decreased catalase activity

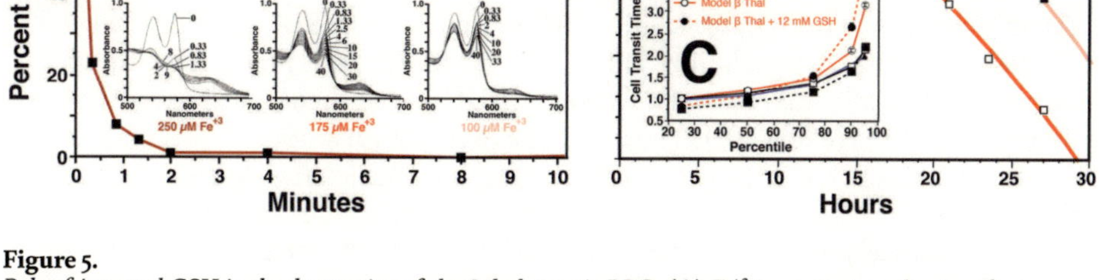

Figure 5.
Role of iron and GSH in the destruction of the β thalassemic RBC. (A) Fe^{+3} is a potent accelerator of hemoglobin oxidation. Shown is the oxyhemoglobin concentration following the addition of 100, 175 and 250 μM Fe^{+3} to a fresh RBC hemolysate. In contrast to the Fe^{+3}-treated samples, no oxidation was observed in the absence of added Fe^{+3} or in the presence of an iron chelator [DFO (deferoxamine) or, not shown, the tripeptide Gly-His-Lys]. Also shown are sequential, hemoglobin scans of the hemolysates treated with Fe^{+3}. The time, in minutes, of the individual scan line following addition of Fe^{+3} are indicated [23, 27]. (B) Depletion of GSH in model β thalassemic RBC inhibits hemoglobin oxidation. Shown is the percent oxyhemoglobin in control-resealed and model β thalassemic cells RBC over 27 h at 37°C. GSH was depleted by treatment with 1-chloro-2.4-dinitrobenzene (CDNB) as previously described [18, 20, 31, 32]. (C) Elevated intracellular GSH levels in model β thalassemic RBC adversely affects cellular deformability as demonstrated by the cell transit analyzer. Less deformable cells take much longer to transit through a pore of known diameter and length. The results shown are the mean ± S.D. of a minimum of four experiments with >2000 RBC measured at each time point. From references: [23, 27].

Population	Hours (37°C)	GSH (μmol/g Hb)	$NADPH/NADP_{total}$ (1.0 = Normal)	Cat. activity (IU/g Hb)
Control RBC	0	5.6 ± 0.4	0.870	147,300 ± 17,000
	20	6.0 ± 0.6	1.063	154,100 ± 14,800
Model β Thal	0	5.2 ± 0.3	0.898	145,600 ± 12,300
	20	2.1 ± 0.0*	0.478*	89,540 ± 8200*

*Modified from [27].*p < 0.001from time-matched Control RBC.*

Table 3.
Association between NADPH, GSH and catalase.

(**Table 3**). Catalase is the pre-eminent defense against H_2O_2 within the RBC, making β thalassemic cell particularly increasingly sensitive to H_2O_2 generated via the pathway described in **Figure 4** [31–34, 43]. Following 20 h incubation at 37°C, only 61.5 ± 2.9% of the initial catalase activity remained in the α-hemoglobin chain loaded cells versus 104.6 ± 4.5% in the control RBC. The loss of catalase arose due to the decrease in the $NADPH/NADP_{total}$ ratio as studies have demonstrated that NADPH is essential for maintaining catalase in an enzymatically active state [31–34, 43–47]. Indeed, as noted in **Table 3**, the model β thalassemic erythrocytes exhibit a significant decrease in the $NADPH/NADP_{total}$ ratio similar to that seen in severe G6PD deficiency. Hence, consequent to the oxidation of hemoglobin and the formation of free radicals in the thalassemic RBC, significant metabolic and functional changes are noted in the model β thalassemic RBC that mirror those seen in patient derived samples (**Figure 4** and **Table 2**). It is also important to note that non-oxidative driven damage also occurs. As shown in **Figure 4**, precipitated globin proteins, as well as iron and heme, can alter the intracellular viscosity of the cytoplasm and interact with the cytoskeleton and membrane lipids resulting in mechanical dysfunction. These oxidative and non-oxidative injuries can dramatically affect the function of the RBC.

4. Loss of RBC deformability and vascular survival

From a functional standpoint, perhaps the most important consequence of the oxidative changes to the β thalassemic RBC, as well as other RBC abnormalities, is the loss of cellular deformability [18–27, 29–33, 48–52]. The physiology, fluidics and vascular bed of the circulatory system impart unique rheological stresses on circulating RBC (**Figure 6A**) [53]. These include extreme variations in shear stress and viscosity as well as biomechanical obstacles (e.g., capillaries and splenic filtration). With an average resting cardiac output of approximately 5 L/min, blood flow varies from approximately 40 cm/s in the aorta to 0.03 cm/s in the smallest capillaries [53, 54]. Moreover, blood viscosity (affecting shear stress) is also variable. At high RBC counts and high flow rates, blood is highly viscous while at low RBC counts and low flow rates (capillaries), blood viscosity is greatly reduced. Rheological stress is further exacerbated by the biomechanical stresses induced by the extreme disparity in the size of RBC (~8 μm) to the minimum diameter of the vascular capillary beds (4–5 μm) and splenic interendothelial clefts (0.5–1.0 μm) [55, 56]. Hence, consequent to the shear forces, viscosity and biomechanical stresses placed on blood cells, a key biologic/physiologic requirement of the RBC within the vascular space is rheological deformability. Biomechanically, the intracellular viscosity and membrane rigidity of the RBC are the key factors in imparting their vascular

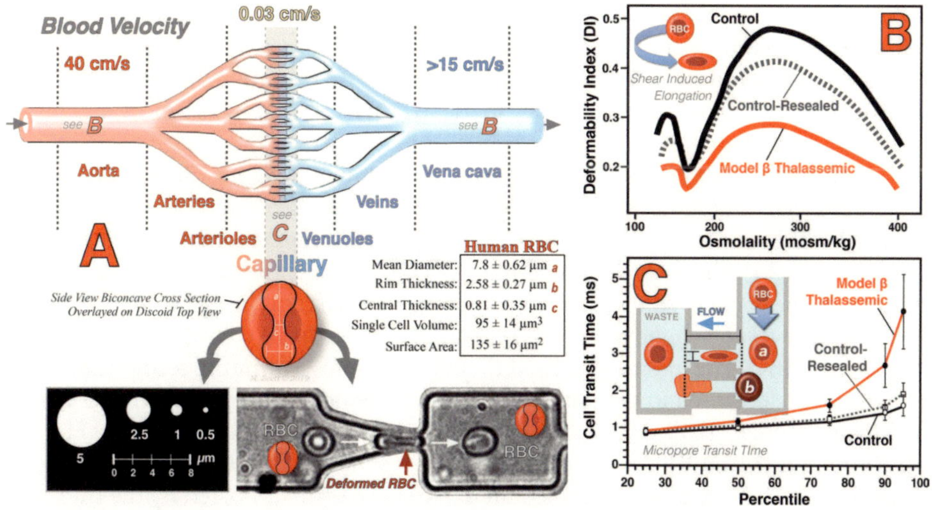

Figure 6.
Vascular deformability of model β thalassemic RBC. (A) The vascular bed is composed of blood vessels of various sizes which create significant disparity in blood (fluid and cellular) velocity consequent to vessel diameter. The fluid flow induces rheological sheer stress while the vessel size creates biomechanical deformation of cellular elements. Shown is an RBC undergoing deformation in a microfluidic channel. (B) Ektacytometric analysis of α-chain loaded RBC demonstrate that these chains dramatically reduce the sheer-induced shape change of the cell [24]. Ektacytometry bests approximates high flow rates. (C) The mean cell transit time (in ms) of model β thalassemic cells was significantly increased, similarly to that observed in patient samples [20]. This microfluidic flow best approximates capillary flow.

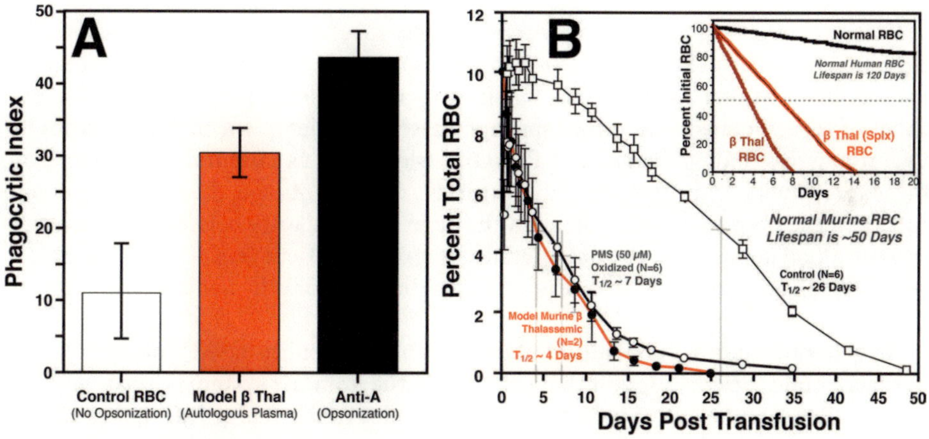

Figure 7.
Model β thalassemic RBC are immunologically recognized and cleared rapidly from the peripheral circulation in vivo. *(A) Blood group A RBC that were loaded with purified α-chains were phagocytosed by human monocytes. Shown for comparison are control cells from the same donor that were either unopsonized or opsonized with an anti-A blood typing antibody. (B) Model β thalassemic mouse RBC were made by the entrapment of purified human α-hemoglobin chains within Normal murine RBC. Oxidatively damaged RBC were made by treating mouse RBC with 50 μM phenazine methosulfate (PMS) for 2.5 h then washing. Both PMS-treatment and the entrapment of α-hemoglobin chains lead to membrane iron deposition and extensive RBC oxidation. The model β thalassemic and PMS-treated RBC have half-lives of 4 and 7 days, respectively in the peripheral circulation versus 26 days for normal murine RBC. Shown is the percent total RBC mass that is PKH-26 labeled. Inset: The peripheral blood lifespan of the human β thalassemic RBC are approximately 6–10 days in a patient with a functioning spleen and 12–16 days in a splenectomized individual. Normal RBC circulates approximately 120 days, data modified from Blendis et al. [69].*

rheological deformability; both of which can be dramatically altered consequent to hemoglobin oxidation, heme release and/or redox-damage to cytoplasmic, cytoskeletal, or membrane components (**Figure 4**) [57–68]. Indeed, as shown in **Figure 6B**, ektacytometric analysis of the model β thalassemic RBC shows a significant loss of cellular deformability induced by shear stress (e.g., large vessels). Moreover, cell transit analysis of these cells (analogous to capillary deformation) showed a very significant loss of deformability in the model β thalassemic cells as reflected by the very large and significant increase in transit time (**Figure 6C**).

Consequent to the loss of deformability and immune recognition (e.g., Kupffer cells of the liver and, potentially, antibodies), the circulatory survival of β thalassemic RBC is impacted. As demonstrated in **Figure 7A**, model β thalassemic RBC (Blood group A) exhibited enhanced immune recognition and phagocytosis by autologous monocytes when compared to control cells from the same donor. Indeed, the level of phagocytosis was similar to that of the anti-A opsonized positive control RBC. The loss of deformability and enhanced immune recognition both contribute to decreased *in vivo* survival. This was demonstrated using mice transfused with model β thalassemic murine cells (mouse RBC + human α-chains) in which the transfused RBC exhibited a dramatic reduction in the circulatory lifespan (**Figure 7B**). The role of α-chain mediated oxidation was supported by the finding that lightly oxidized (phenazine methosulphate treated; 50 μM) murine cells showed similar circulatory dynamics. These results are comparable to that observed in humans where, consequent to the α-chain driven oxidation, β thalassemic RBC have a very short circulatory lifespan (7–14 days depending on spleen status) compared to the 120 days of a normal RBC.

5. Immunological dysfunction: Effect on antigen presentation

Interestingly, thalassemias have been clinically associated with an increased risk of recurrent bacterial infections [70–87]. This is most evident in under-developed nations where sanitary and medical facilities are most lacking. Despite the clinical evidence of recurrent bacterial infections in thalassemic patients, the biological events underlying this finding are unclear. This confusion arises as a natural consequence of the heterogeneity of the microbial disease itself, the patients age, the state of splenic function, the frequency of transfusion, the degree of similarity between the patient and the blood donor pool, the nutritional status of the patient (e.g., United States versus Thailand) and whether one is looking at humoral or cell-mediated immunity [70–87].

In general, studies on the humoral (i.e., immunoglobulin-based) immunity of thalassemic patients suggest that this arm of the immune system is 'relatively' normal. These studies have indicated normal to elevated levels of IgG, IgA, and IgM but decreased levels of Factor B, C3, and C4 (perhaps due to consumption via oxidatively damaged β thalassemic cells). Reflective of this normality, and consequent to the extensive oxidant injury to the thalassemic cells, circulating immune complexes and an elevated risk of autoimmune hemolytic anemia have been described in β thalassemia intermedia and major patients. Serum fractions from these patients also exhibited increased amounts of C1q-precipitable immune complexes. In contrast, as suggested by the clinically described recurrent bacterial infections, cell-mediated immunity is highly suspect in the thalassemic patient (and sickle cell patients). The few direct studies on cell-mediated immunity in thalassemic patients were, typically, enumeration of the mononuclear cell populations (T cells, B cells, NK cells and monocytes). In general, these studies suggest normal cell numbers but a skewed distribution of the $CD4^+$ to $CD8^+$ T cell ratio. The altered ratio was characterized by a relative depression in $CD4^+$ T cells (i.e., helper T cells) and NK (Natural Killer) cells and a relative rise in $CD8^+$ (cytotoxic and suppressor) T cells that increased linearly with the number of units transfused. However, very few functional studies have been done in thalassemic patients to answer the question: *Why are β thalassemic patients at risk of recurrent bacterial infections?*

Previous studies have suggested that increased bioavailable iron in transfused patients might facilitate the growth of organisms in which iron is a limiting nutrient (i.e., most bacteria). Other studies have implicated the loss of splenic function. While both of these factors may indeed play important roles in recurrent bacterial infections, they may not offer a complete explanation. In addition to thalassemia, a number of other diseases and trauma scenarios are characterized by recurrent bacterial infections (e.g., malaria and burn injury) suggestive of impaired cell-mediated immunity. Interestingly, a common characteristic of all these conditions is erythrophagocytosis. Previous studies have demonstrated that phagocytic uptake of IgG-coated and oxidatively stressed RBC resulted in a transient depression of further macrophage phagocytosis, decreased respiratory burst (i.e., NADPH-oxidase activity; O_2^- production), and impaired killing of bacteria [88–93]. Interestingly, in the case of *Plasmodium falciparum*-infected RBC, only phagocytosis of mature (trophozoite), but not immature (ring stage), stages had an inhibitory effect on monocyte function. Importantly, a major difference between the mature and immature malarial infected RBC is the presence of malarial pigment (hemozoin), an iron/heme rich degradation product of parasite hemoglobin catabolism. The heme- and iron-rich membranes of the β thalassemic RBC, which we have previously documented [22], may function in a manner analogous to malarial pigment or iron salts and impair cell-mediated immunity—primarily at the level of the APC but potentially extending to the T cell level. Some data from thalassemic patients support the hypothesis for impairment of the T cell response. For example, patients with thalassemia intermedia have been reported to have diminished T cell mitogen responses when their serum iron and ferritin were higher than 200 and 600 μg/dl, respectively [94].

Hence, injury arising from the iron-GSH pathway can result in (any combination of) RBC opsonization by endogenous antibodies, phosphatidylserine (PS) exposure, protein clustering, sublytic levels of complement binding, and/or loss of cellular deformability (**Figure 7**) that leads to the removal of the damaged β thalassemic cells from the circulatory system by components of the mononuclear phagocytic system (MPS). Erythrophagocytosis can occur within the spleen (if present and functioning), liver (Kupffer cells) or the microvasculature itself when

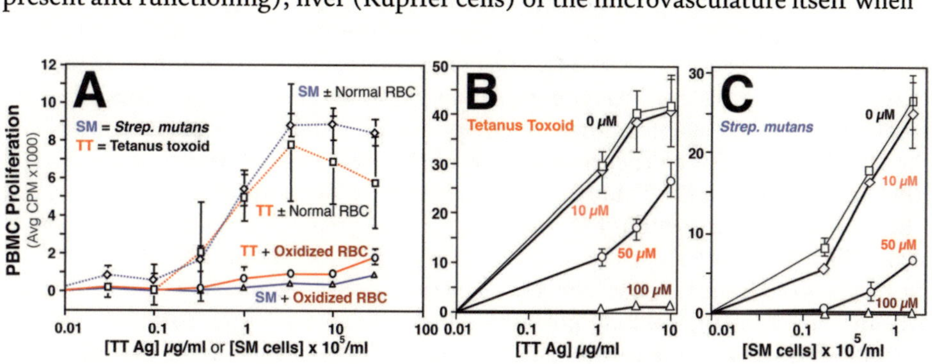

Figure 8.
Antigen processing and presentation is inhibited by oxidized RBC and hemin. (A) Antigen presentation of TT and SM was inhibited by the erythrophagocytosis of oxidized RBC. Normal RBC had no inhibitory effect. The efficacy of antigen processing and/or presentation was assessed by ^{3}H-thymidine incorporation in proliferating T cells. PBMC were resuspended in Aim V media at a final concentration of 2.5 × 10^5 PBMC per 200 μl. Final RBC concentration was 8 × 10^6 per 200 μl. Antigens were diluted in Aim V and added at the indicated concentrations. Results shown are of a representative experiment with quadruplicate samples. (B, C) Heme pretreatment of PBMC (2 h at 37°C) dramatically inhibits the proliferative response to tetanus toxoid (B) and S. mutans *(C). Interestingly, the ability of PBMC to respond to intact bacteria is more significantly blunted than is the response to tetanus toxoid at intermediate hemin concentrations (50 μM). Results shown are of a representative experiment with quadruplicate samples.*

non-deformable RBC are trapped and then cleared by circulating macrophages. Regardless of the location of removal, erythrophagocytosis results in impaired MPS function. As shown in **Figure 8A**, antigen presentation of purified tetanus toxoid (TT; a peptide) or fixed, intact, *S. mutans* (SM; an intact bacteria) by normal human antigen presenting cells (APC; blood monocytes) was dramatically, and differentially, affected by the presence of either control (unoxidized) or oxidized (50 μM PMS as per **Figure 7**) human RBC. As shown, oxidized RBC prevented successful antigen presentation to human T cells while normal RBC showed no detrimental effects. Further experimentation demonstrated that the inhibitory effect was due to heme/iron. As shown in **Figure 8B, C**, direct addition of hemin to the APC impaired successful antigen presentation of both tetanus toxoid and Strep. mutans in a dose dependent manner.

6. Conclusions

β thalassemias arise from a number of underlying genetic defects that interfere with the synthesis of the β hemoglobin chain and the subsequent production of the normal $\alpha_2\beta_2$ hemoglobin tetramer. As a consequence of this decreased/absent β-chain synthesis, unpaired, monomeric, α-hemoglobin chains are produced. While the presence of the highly unstable α-chains mediate the pathophysiology of the RBC, it has been difficult to fully elucidate the mechanisms underlying their destructive processes in human cells. This lack of understanding of the mechanisms of α-chain mediated damage is due, in large part, to the fact that peripheral RBC isolated from β thalassemic individuals are already severely damaged cells (with most being destroyed within the bone marrow). Moreover, severe β thalassemia patients are typically transfused to both correct the severe anemia accompanying the disease and to prevent endogenous erythropoiesis of defective RBC. Hence, murine models of β thalassemia have been developed and extensively studied. However, problems exist with these models (e.g., mouse vs. human α-chains; interaction of human globins with mouse cytoskeletal proteins) and these mice, as in human patients, still suffer from the heterogeneity of RBC changes arising from the different ages of the peripheral blood RBC [11–17].

To better study the *fate of unpaired α-chains* in human RBC, the model β thalassemic cell was developed [18–34]. The entrapment of purified α-hemoglobin chains within normal erythrocytes via osmotic lysis and resealing provides an excellent and reproducible human model for studying the pathologic effects of the unpaired α-chains on the structural and functional characteristics of the RBC. Indeed, as noted in **Table 2**, the α-chain induced structural and functional RBC changes are very similar to those observed in human donor derived β thalassemic RBC. Schematically the pathophysiology of the β thalassemic RBC, and its downstream consequences, as elucidated by the model human β thalassemic RBC, are summarized in **Figure 9**. Importantly, these studies have demonstrated that the unpaired α-chains initiate an *iron, GSH-dependent, self-amplifying and self-propagating reaction* with the subsequent release of even more heme and, eventually, free iron (**Figure 4**). Membrane proteins and reactive thiol groups (not shown) were rapidly decreased in a pattern similar to that observed *in vivo* in β thalassemia [18, 20–23, 25–27]. These oxidative events also result in membrane vesiculation of the thalassemic RBC. One consequence of membrane vesiculation is the preferential loss of phosphatidylinositol (PI) anchored proteins from the RBC. Among these PI-anchored proteins are decay accelerating factor (DAF; CD55) and the membrane inhibitor of reactive lysis (MIRL; CD59) both of which play important roles in preventing complement-mediated binding and lysis. The effects of the

DOI: http://dx.doi.org/10.5772/intechopen.90288

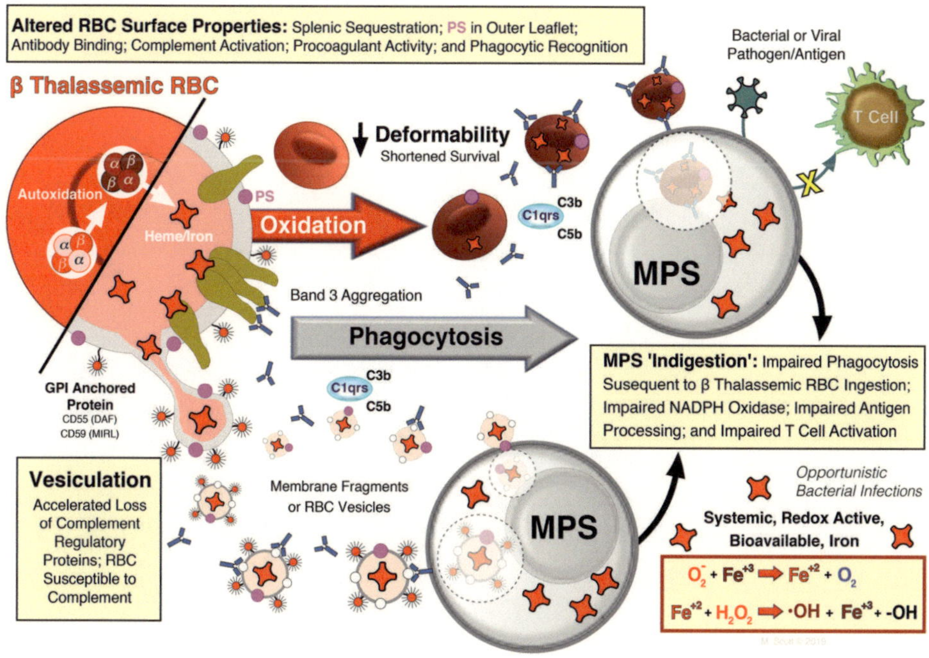

Figure 9.
Schematic representation of the pathophysiology of the β thalassemic RBC and its immunological consequences.

vesiculation-mediated loss of CD55 and CD59 can range from sublytic levels of bound complement enhancing phagocytosis to overt hemolysis. Indeed, a common endpoint for all the α-chain mediated injury is enhanced erythrophagocytosis. As shown, oxidized RBC or the heme from these cells (**Figure 8**) significantly inhibits antigen processing, presentation and T cell proliferation. The systemic importance of this on cell-mediated immunity has not be fully appreciated and may potentially explain the predisposition of thalassemic patients to recurrent bacterial infections.

In sum, these findings show the utility of the model β thalassemic human RBC for investigating the pathophysiology of the unpaired α-chains. Moreover, these cells are easily 'manufactured' from normal donor RBC and may provide an effective means to evaluate therapeutic approaches to ameliorate the damage to the thalassemic cell in β thalassemia intermedia in order to prolong RBC survival and reduce transfusions [23, 25–27, 40].

Acknowledgements

This work was supported by grants from Canadian Blood Services and Health Canada. The views expressed herein do not necessarily represent the view of the federal government of Canada. We thank the Canada Foundation for Innovation and the Michael Smith Foundation for Health Research for infrastructure funding at the University of British Columbia Centre for Blood Research. The funders had no role in study design, data collection and analysis, decision to publish, or preparation of the manuscript.

Conflict of interest

There are no conflicts of interest.

Author details

Mark D. Scott[1,2,3]

1 Canadian Blood Services, Ottawa, ON, Canada

2 Centre for Blood Research, University of British Columbia, Vancouver, BC, Canada

3 Department of Pathology and Laboratory Medicine, University of British Columbia, Vancouver, BC, Canada

*Address all correspondence to: mdscott@mail.ubc.ca

References

[1] Robinson AR, Robson M, Harrison AP, Zuelzer WW. A new technique for differentiation of hemoglobin. The Journal of Laboratory and Clinical Medicine. 1957;**50**:745-752. PMID: 13476032

[2] Weatherall DJ, Clegg JB. Molecular basis of thalassemia. British Journal of Haematology. 1975;**31**:133-141. DOI: 10.1111/j.1365-2141.1975.tb00906.x

[3] Weatherall DJ. Pathophysiology of thalassaemia. Baillière's Clinical Haematology. 1998;**11**:127-146. PMID: 10872475

[4] Higgs DR. The molecular basis of α-thalassemia. Cold Spring Harbor Perspectives in Medicine. 2013;**3**:a011718. DOI: 10.1101/cshperspect.a011718

[5] Piel FB, Weatherall DJ. The α-thalassemias. The New England Journal of Medicine. 2014;**371**:1908-1916. DOI: 10.1056/NEJMra1404415

[6] Mettananda S, Gibbons RJ, Higgs DR. α-Globin as a molecular target in the treatment of β-thalassemia. Blood. 2015;**125**:3694-3701. DOI: 10.1182/blood-2015-03-633594

[7] Mettananda S, Higgs DR. Molecular basis and genetic modifiers of thalassemia. Hematology/Oncology Clinics of North America. 2018;**32**:177-191. DOI: 10.1016/j.hoc.2017.11.003

[8] Taher AT, Weatherall DJ, Cappellini MD. Thalassaemia. Lancet. 2018;**391**:155-167. DOI: 10.1016/S0140-6736(17)31822-6

[9] Weatherall DJ. The evolving spectrum of the epidemiology of thalassemia. Hematology/Oncology Clinics of North America. 2018;**32**:165-175. DOI: 10.1016/j.hoc.2017.11.008

[10] Turbpaiboon C, Wilairat P. Alpha-hemoglobin stabilizing protein: Molecular function and clinical correlation. Frontiers in Bioscience (Landmark Edition). 2010;**15**:1-11. PMID: 20036801

[11] Rubin EM, Kan YW, Mohandas N. Effect of human beta (s)-globin chains on cellular properties of red cells from beta-thalassemic mice. The Journal of Clinical Investigation. 1988;**82**:1129-1133. DOI: 10.1172/JCI113670

[12] Sorensen S, Rubin E, Polster H, Mohandas N, Schrier S. The role of membrane skeletal-associated alpha-globin in the pathophysiology of beta-thalassemia. Blood. 1990;**75**:1333-1336. PMID: 1690033

[13] Advani R, Rubin E, Mohandas N, Schrier SL. Oxidative red blood cell membrane injury in the pathophysiology of severe mouse β-thalassemias. Blood. 1992;**79**:1064-1067. PMID: 1737090

[14] Pászty C. Transgenic and gene knock-out mouse models of sickle cell anemia and the thalassemias. Current Opinion in Hematology. 1997;**4**:88-93. PMID: 9107524

[15] Nishino T, Cao H, Stamatoyannopoulos G, Emery DW. Effects of human gamma-globin in murine beta-thalassaemia. British Journal of Haematology. 2006;**134**:100-108. DOI: 10.1111/j.1365-2141.2006.06102.x

[16] Huo Y, McConnell SC, Liu SR, Yang R, Zhang TT, Sun CW, et al. Humanized mouse model of Cooley's anemia. The Journal of Biological Chemistry. 2009;**284**:4889-4896. DOI: 10.1074/jbc.M805681200

[17] McColl B, Vadolas J. Animal models of β-hemoglobinopathies: Utility and

limitations. Journal of Blood Medicine. 2016;7:263-274. DOI: 10.2147/JBM.S87955

[18] Scott MD, Rouyer-Fessard P, Lubin BH, Beuzard Y. Entrapment of purified alpha-hemoglobin chains in normal erythrocytes. A model for beta thalassemia. Journal of Biological Chemistry. 1990;**265**:17953-17959. PMID: 2211672

[19] Rouyer-Fessard P, Scott MD, Leroy-Viard K, Garel MC, Bachir D, Galacteros F, et al. Fate of alpha-hemoglobin chains and erythrocyte defects in beta-thalassemia. Annals of the New York Academy of Sciences. 1990;**612**:106-117. DOI: 10.1111/j.1749-6632.1990.tb24296.x

[20] Scott MD, Rouyer-Fessard P, Ba MS, Lubin BH, Beuzard Y. Alpha- and beta-haemoglobin chain induced changes in normal erythrocyte deformability: Comparison to beta thalassaemia intermedia and Hb H disease. British Journal of Haematology. 1992;**80**:519-526. DOI: 10.1111/j.1365-2141.1992.tb04567.x

[21] Scott MD. Entrapment of purified alpha-hemoglobin chains in normal erythrocytes as a model for human beta thalassemia. Advances in Experimental Medicine and Biology. 1992;**326**:139-148. PMID: 1295299

[22] Scott MD, van den Berg JJ, Repka T, Rouyer-Fessard P, Hebbel RP, Beuzard Y, et al. Effect of excess alpha-hemoglobin chains on cellular and membrane oxidation in model beta-thalassemic erythrocytes. The Journal of Clinical Investigation. 1993;**91**:1706-1712. DOI: 10.1172/JCI116380

[23] Scott MD, Eaton JW. Thalassaemic erythrocytes: Cellular suicide arising from iron and glutathione-dependent oxidation reactions? British Journal of Haematology. 1995;**91**:811-819. DOI: 10.1111/j.1365-2141.1995.tb05394.x

[24] Kuypers FA, Schott MA, Scott MD. Phospholipid composition and organization in model beta-thalassemic erythrocytes. American Journal of Hematology. 1996;**51**:45-54. DOI: 10.1002/(SICI)1096-8652(199601)51:1<45::AID-AJH8>3.0.CO;2-7

[25] Scott MD, Yang L, Ulrich P, Shupe T. Pharmacologic interception of heme: A potential therapeutic strategy for the treatment of ß thalassemia? Redox Report. 1997;**3**:159-167. DOI: 10.1080/13510002.1997.11747104

[26] Scott MD. Intraerythrocytic iron chelation: A new therapy for thalassemia. Hematology. 2001;**6**:73-89. DOI: 10.1080/10245332.2001.11746557

[27] Scott MD. H_2O_2 injury in beta thalassemic erythrocytes: Protective role of catalase and the prooxidant effects of GSH. Free Radical Biology & Medicine. 2006;**40**:1264-1272. DOI: 10.1016/j.freeradbiomed.2005.11.017

[28] Scott MD, Eaton JW, Kuypers FA, Chiu D-Y, Lubin BH. Enhancement of erythrocyte superoxide dismutase activity: Effects on cellular oxidant defense. Blood. 1989;**74**:2542-2549. PMID: 2553167

[29] Scott MD, Kuypers FA, Butikofer P, Bookchin RM, Ortiz OE, Lubin BH. Effect of osmotic lysis and resealing on red cell structure and function. The Journal of Laboratory and Clinical Medicine. 1990;**115**:470-480. PMID: 1691257

[30] Scott MD, Ranz A, Kuypers FA, Lubin BH, Meshnick SR. Parasite uptake of desferroxamine: A prerequisite for antimalarial activity. British Journal of Haematology. 1990;**75**:598-602. DOI: 10.1111/j.1365-2141.1990.tb07805.x

[31] Scott MD, Lubin BH, Zuo L, Kuypers FA. Erythrocyte defense

against hydrogen peroxide: Preeminent importance of catalase. The Journal of Laboratory and Clinical Medicine. 1991;**118**:7-16. PMID: 2066646

[32] Scott MD, Zuo L, Lubin BH, Chiu DT. NADPH, not glutathione, status modulates oxidant sensitivity in normal and glucose-6-phosphate dehydrogenase-deficient erythrocytes. Blood. 1991;**77**:2059-2064. PMID: 2018843

[33] Scott MD, Wagner TC, Chiu DT. Decreased catalase activity is the underlying mechanism of oxidant susceptibility in glucose-6-phosphate dehydrogenase-deficient erythrocytes. Biochimica et Biophysica Acta. 1993;**1181**:163-168. DOI: 10.1016/0925-4439(93)90106-b

[34] Scott MD. Glucose-6-phosphate dehydrogenase deficiency: A new hypothesis for an old disease. Redox Report. 1995;**1**:235-237. DOI: 10.1080/13510002.1995.11746992

[35] Bucci E, Fronticelli C. A new method for the preparation of alpha and beta subunits of human hemoglobin. The Journal of Biological Chemistry. 1965;**240**:PC551-PC552. PMID: 14253474

[36] Abraham EC, Reese A, Stallings M, Huisman TH. Separation of human hemoglobins by DEAE-cellulose chromatography using glycine-KCN-NaC1 developers. Hemoglobin. 1976;**1**:27-44. PMID: 1052169

[37] Bunn HF, Jandl JH. Exchange of heme among hemoglobins and between hemoglobin and albumin. The Journal of Biological Chemistry. 1968;**243**:465-475. PMID: 4966113

[38] Brunori M, Falcioni G, Fioretti E, Giardina B, Rotilio G. Formation of superoxide in the autoxidation of the isolated α and β chains of human hemoglobin and its involvement in hemichrome precipitation. European Journal of Biochemistry. 1975;**53**:99-104. DOI: 10.1111/j.1432-1033.1975.tb04046.x

[39] Joshi W, Leb L, Piotrowski J, Fortier N, Snyder LM. Increased sensitivity of isolated alpha subunits of normal human hemoglobin to oxidative damage and crosslinking with spectrin. The Journal of Laboratory and Clinical Medicine. 1983;**102**:46-52. PMID: 6854133

[40] Rossi NA, Mustafa I, Jackson JK, Burt HM, Horte SA, Scott MD, et al. In vitro chelating, cytotoxicity, and blood compatibility of degradable poly(ethylene glycol)-based macromolecular iron chelators. Biomaterials. 2009;**30**:638-648. DOI: 10.1016/j.biomaterials.2008.09.057

[41] Lunn G, Dale GL, Beutler E. Transport accounts for glutathione turnover in human erythrocytes. Blood. 1979;**54**:238-244. PMID: 444668

[42] Raftos JE, Whillier S, Kuchel PW. Glutathione synthesis and turnover in the human erythrocyte: Alignment of a model based on detailed enzyme kinetics with experimental data. The Journal of Biological Chemistry. 2010;**285**:23557-23567. DOI: 10.1074/jbc.M109.067017

[43] Wagner TC, Scott MD. Single extraction method for the spectrophotometric quantification of oxidized and reduced pyridine nucleotides in erythrocytes. Analytical Biochemistry. 1994;**222**:417-426. DOI: 10.1006/abio.1994.1511

[44] Eaton JW, Boraas M, Etkin NL. Catalase activity and red cell metabolism. In: Brewer GJ, editor. Hemoglobin and Red Cell Structure and Function. New York: Plenum Publishing Corp; 1972. pp. 121-131. DOI: 10.1007/978-1-4684-3222-0_8

[45] Kirkman HN, Gaetani GF. Catalase: A tetrameric enzyme with four tightly bound molecules of NADPH. Proceedings of the National Academy of Sciences of the United States of America. 1984;**81**:4343-4347. DOI: 10.1073/pnas.81.14.4343

[46] Kirkman HN, Galiano S, Gaetani GF. The function of catalase-bound NADPH. The Journal of Biological Chemistry. 1987;**262**:660-666. PMID: 3805001

[47] Gaetani GF, Canepa L, Galiano S, Ferraris AM, Kirkman HK. Catalase and glutathione peroxidase are equally active in the detoxification of hydrogen peroxide in human erythrocytes. Blood. 1989;**73**:334-339. PMID: 2491951

[48] Scott MD, Meshnick SR, Williams RA, Chiu DT, Pan HC, Lubin BH, et al. Qinghaosu-mediated oxidation in normal and abnormal erythrocytes. The Journal of Laboratory and Clinical Medicine. 1989;**114**:401-406. PMID: 2794752

[49] Meshnick SR, Scott MD, Lubin B, Ranz A, Eaton JW. Antimalarial activity of diethyldithiocarbamate. Potentiation by copper. Biochemical Pharmacology. 1990;**40**:213-216. DOI: 10.1016/0006-2952(90)90680-J

[50] Kuypers FA, Scott MD, Schott MA, Lubin B, Chiu DT. Use of ektacytometry to determine red cell susceptibility to oxidative stress. The Journal of Laboratory and Clinical Medicine. 1990;**116**:535-545. PMID: 2212862

[51] Hong YL, Pan HZ, Scott MD, Meshnick SR. Activated oxygen generation by a primaquine metabolite: Inhibition by antioxidants derived from Chinese herbal remedies. Free Radical Biology & Medicine. 1992;**12**:213-218. DOI: 10.1016/0891-5849(92)90029-G

[52] Minetti M, Mallozzi C, Scorza G, Scott MD, Kuypers FA, Lubin BH. Role of oxygen and carbon radicals in hemoglobin oxidation. Archives of Biochemistry and Biophysics. 1993;**302**:233-244. DOI: 10.1006/abbi.1993.1205

[53] Aird WC. Spatial and temporal dynamics of the endothelium. Journal of Thrombosis and Haemostasis. 2005;**3**:1392-1406. DOI: 10.1111/j.1538-7836.2005.01328.x

[54] Wexler L, Bergel DH, Gabe IT, Makin GS, Mills CJ. Velocity of blood flow in normal human venae cavae. Circulation Research. 1968;**23**:349-359. DOI: 10.1161/01.RES.23.3.349

[55] Weiss L, Tavassoli M. Anatomical hazards to the passage of erythrocytes through the spleen. Seminars in Hematology. 1970;7:372-380. PMID: 5473419

[56] Chen LT, Weiss L. The role of the sinus wall in the passage of erythrocytes through the spleen. Blood. 1973;**41**:529-537. PMID: 4688868

[57] LaCelle PL. Alteration of membrane deformability in hemolytic anemias. Seminars in Hematology. 1970;7:355-371. PMID: 5473418

[58] Weed RI. The importance of erythrocyte deformability. The American Journal of Medicine. 1970;**49**:147-150. DOI: 10.1016/S0002-9343(70)80069-9

[59] Chien S, Usami S, Bertles JF. Abnormal rheology of oxygenated blood in sickle cell anemia. The Journal of Clinical Investigation. 1970;**49**:623-634. DOI: 10.1172/JCI106273

[60] Chien S, Usami S, Dellenback RJ, Gregersen MI. Shear-dependent deformation of erythrocytes in rheology of human blood. The American Journal of Physiology. 1970;**219**:136-142. DOI: 10.1152/ajplegacy.1970.219.1.136

[61] Bessis M, Mohandas N. Red cell structure, shapes and deformability. British Journal of Haematology. 1975;**31**:5-11. DOI: 10.1111/j.1365-2141.1975.tb00893.x

[62] La Celle PL. Pathogenic erythrocytes in the capillary microcirculation. Blood Cells. 1975;**1**:269-284

[63] Havell TC, Hillman D, Lessin LS. Deformability characteristics of sickle cells by microelastimetry. American Journal of Hematology. 1978;**4**:9-16. DOI: 10.1002/ajh.2830040103

[64] Mohandas N, Phillips WM, Bessis M. Red blood cell deformability and hemolytic anemias. Seminars in Hematology. 1979;**16**:95-114. PMID: 384522

[65] Clark MR, Mohandas N, Shohet SB. Deformability of oxygenated irreversibly sickled cells. The Journal of Clinical Investigation. 1980;**65**:189-195. DOI: 10.1172/JCI109650

[66] Clark MR, Mohandas N, Shohet SB. Osmotic gradient ektacytometry: Comprehensive characterization of red cell volume and surface maintenance. Blood. 1983;**61**:899-910. PMID: 6831052

[67] Snyder LM, Fortier NL, Trainor J, Jacobs J, Leb L, Lubin B, et al. Effect of hydrogen peroxide exposure on normal human erythrocyte deformability, morphology, surface characteristics, and spectrin-hemoglobin cross-linking. The Journal of Clinical Investigation. 1985;**76**:1971-1977. DOI: 10.1172/JCI112196

[68] Snyder LM, Fortier NL, Leb L, McKenney J, Trainor J, Sheerin H, et al. The role of membrane protein sulfhydryl groups in hydrogen peroxide-mediated membrane damage in human erythrocytes. Biochimica et Biophysica Acta. 1988;**937**:229-240. DOI: 10.1016/0005-2736(88)90245-3

[69] Blendis LM, Modell CB, Bowdler AJ, Williams R. Some effects of splenectomy in thalassaemia major. British Journal of Haematology. 1974;**28**:77-87. DOI: 10.1111/j.1365-2141.1974.tb06641.x

[70] Dickerman JD. Bacterial infection and the asplenic host: A review. The Journal of Trauma. 1976;**16**:662-668. DOI: 10.1097/00005373-197608000-00012

[71] Dickerman JD. Splenectomy and sepsis: A warning. Pediatrics. 1979;**63**:938-941. PMID: 377203

[72] Borgna-Pignatti C, De Stefano P, Barone F, Concia E. Penicillin compliance in splenectomized thalassemics. European Journal of Pediatrics. 1984;**142**:83-85. PMID: 6468437

[73] Fucharoen S, Piankijagum A, Wasi P. Deaths in beta-thalassemia/Hb E patients secondary to infections. Birth Defects Original Article Series. 1987;**23**:495-500. PMID: 3689937

[74] Aswapokee P, Aswapokee N, Fucharoen S, Sukroongreung S, Wasi P. Severe infection in thalassemia: A prospective study. Birth Defects Original Article Series. 1987;**23**:521-526. PMID: 3689941

[75] Wasi C, Kuntang R, Louisirirotchanakul S, Siritantikorn S, Fucharoen S, Aswapokee P, et al. Viral infections in beta-thalassemia/hemoglobin E patients. Birth Defects Original Article Series. 1987;**23**:547-555. PMID: 2825835

[76] Swarup-Mitra S. Immunologic status of Hb E-thalassemia patients. Birth Defects. 1988;**23**:571-579. PMID: 3689944

[77] Swarup-Mitra S. Morbidity pattern in Hb E-thalassemia disease. Birth Defects Original Article Series. 1988;**23**:501-504. PMID: 3689938

[78] Sukroongreung S, Nilakul C, Aswapokee N, Aswapokee P, Fucharoen S, Wasi P. Oropharyngeal colonization with aerobic bacteria in β-thalassemia/hemoglobin E disease. Birth Defects Original Article Series. 1988;**23**:535-541. PMID: 3318952

[79] Sukroongreung S, Wasi P. Serum of thalassemic patients promotes growth of *Streptococci*. Birth Defects Original Article Series. 1988;**23**:543-546. PMID: 3689943

[80] Ampel NM, Van Wyck DB, Aguirre ML, Willis DG, Popp RA. Resistance to infection in murine beta-thalassemia. Infection and Immunity. 1989;**57**:1011-1017. PMCID: PMC313221

[81] Ampel NM, Bejarano GC, Saavedra M. Deferoxamine increases the susceptibility of beta-thalassemic, iron-overloaded mice to infection with Listeria monocytogenes. Life Sciences. 1992;**50**:1327-1332. DOI: 10.1016/0024-3205(92)90283-u

[82] Cherchi GB, Cossellu S, Pacifico L, Gallisai D, Ranucci A, Zanetti S, et al. Incidence and outcome of *Yersinia enterocolitica* infection in thalassemic patients. Contributions to Microbiology and Immunology. 1995;**13**:16-18. PMID: 8833786

[83] Wanachiwanawin W, Phucharoen J, Pattanapanyasat K, Fucharoen S, Webster HK. Lymphocytes in beta-thalassemia/HbE: Subpopulations and mitogen responses. European Journal of Haematology. 1996;**56**:153-157. PMID: 8598234

[84] Vento S, Cainelli F, Cesario F. Infections and thalassaemia. The Lancet Infectious Diseases. 2006;**6**:226-233. DOI: 10.1016/S1473-3099(06)70437-6

[85] Rahav G, Volach V, Shapiro M, Rund D, Rachmilewitz EA, Goldfarb A. Severe infections in thalassaemic patients: Prevalence and predisposing factors. British Journal of Haematology. 2006;**133**:667-674. DOI: 10.1111/j.1365-2141.2006.06082.x

[86] Yapp AR, Lindeman R, Gilroy N, Gao Z, Macintyre CR. Infection outcomes in splenectomized patients with hemoglobinopathies in Australia. International Journal of Infectious Diseases. 2009;**13**:696-700. DOI: 10.1016/j.ijid.2008.10.011

[87] Kao JK, Wang SC, Ho LW, Huang SW, Chang SH, Yang RC, et al. Chronic Iron overload results in impaired bacterial killing of THP-1 derived macrophage through the inhibition of lysosomal acidification. PLoS One. 2016;**11**:e0156713. DOI: 10.1371/journal.pone.0156713

[88] Loegering DJ, Grover GJ, Schneidkraut MJ. Effect of red blood cells and red blood cell ghosts on reticuloendothelial system function. Experimental and Molecular Pathology. 1984;**41**:67-73. DOI: 10.1016/0014-4800(84)90008-X

[89] Loegering DJ, Blumenstock FA. Depressing hepatic macrophage complement receptor function causes increased susceptibility to endotoxemia and infection. Infection and Immunity. 1985;**47**:659-664. PMCID: PMC261348

[90] Commins LM, Loegering DJ, Gudewicz PW. Effect of phagocytosis of erythrocytes and erythrocyte ghosts on macrophage phagocytic function and hydrogen peroxide production. Inflammation. 1990;**14**:705-716. DOI: 10.1007/BF00916373

[91] Loegering DJ, Schwacha MG. Macrophage hydrogen peroxide production and phagocytic function and decreased following phagocytosis mediated by Fc receptors but not complement receptors. Biochemical and Biophysical Research Communications. 1991;**180**:268-272. DOI: 10.1016/S0006-291X(05)81287-2

[92] Schwacha MG, Gudewicz PW, Snyder JA, Loegering DJ. Depression of macrophage respiratory burst capacity and arachidonic acid release after Fc receptor-mediated phagocytosis. Journal of Immunology. 1993;**150**:236-245. PMID: 8417125

[93] Loegering DJ, Raley MJ, Reho TA, Eaton JW. Macrophage dysfunction following the phagocytosis of IgG coated erythrocytes: Production of lipid peroxidation products. Journal of Leukocyte Biology. 1996;**59**:357-363. DOI: 10.1002/jlb.59.3.357

[94] de Sousa M. Blood transfusions and allograft survival: Iron-related immunosuppression [Letter]. Lancet. 1983;**2**(8351):681-682. DOI: 10.1016/s0140-6736(83)92558-8

Chapter 6

Oxidative Stress and Iron Overload in β-Thalassemia: An Overview

Nadia Maria Sposi

Abstract

In β-thalassemia, the erythropoietic process is markedly altered, and the lack or reduced synthesis of β-globin chains induces an excess of free α-globin chains within the erythroid cells. Aggregation, denaturation, and degradation of these chains lead to the formation of insoluble precipitates causing damage to the red blood cell membrane. One of the major consequences in this genetic disorder is iron overload due to ineffective erythropoiesis and premature hemolysis in the plasma and in major organs such as heart, liver, and endocrine glands. The chapter describes the etiology of iron accumulation, the role of hepcidin in regulating increased iron absorption, and the pathophysiology resulting from excess of "free iron" and discusses new ways to decrease the iron overload and to neutralize its deleterious effects in the tissues other than iron chelation.

Keywords: oxidative stress, iron overload, β-thalassemia

1. Introduction

β-thalassemias are a group of hereditary blood disorders characterized by the reduced or absent synthesis of β-globin chains representing one of the most common autosomal recessive disorders worldwide. It is prevalent in the Mediterranean countries, the Middle East, and Southeast Asia, as well as countries along the Americas, coincidental with the occurrence of malaria. Carriers of β-thalassemia genes are considered relatively protected against malaria parasite. At present, because of vast population migration and intermarriage between different ethnic groups, β-thalassemia is also common in North and South America, Northern Europa, Australia, and the Caribbean. As a consequence of the reduced or absent synthesis of β-globin chains, there is an excess on α-globin chains that are instable and precipitate in red blood cell precursors causing abnormal cell maturation and their premature destruction in the bone marrow (ineffective erythropoiesis). Red blood cells that survive to reach the peripheral circulation are prematurely destroyed in the spleen. The break down products of Hb, heme, and iron catalyze chemical reactions that generate free radicals, including reactive oxygen species (ROS), which in excess are toxic, causing damage to vital organs such as the heart and liver and the endocrine system [1]. More than 300 different point mutations cause β-thalassemia. They are inherited in a multitude of genetic combinations responsible for clinical manifestations extremely diverse, spanning a broad spectrum from the transfusion-dependent state of thalassemia major (TM) to the asymptomatic state of heterozygous carriers for β^0 or β^+ (thalassemia trait). β-thalassemia intermedia requires only periodic blood transfusion,

IntechOpen

while β-thalassemia minor does not require a specific treatment. One of the major consequences in this genetic disorder is iron overload due to multiple blood transfusions, ineffective erythropoiesis, and premature hemolysis in the plasma. Cardiomyopathy is the most common cause of death in transfusion-dependent thalassemia patients as a consequence of iron overloading. Thanks to the significant improvement in therapy, patients with β-thalassemia may reach an advanced age. This is associated with clinical symptoms that are the consequence of the disease itself and the treatment modalities. The aim of this chapter is that to give a complete picture of current knowledge on the etiology of iron accumulation, the role of hepcidin in regulating increased iron absorption, and the pathophysiology resulting from excess of "free iron." It will also be explored whether there are ways to decrease the iron overload and to neutralize its deleterious effects in the tissues other than iron chelation (for an extensive revision, see Refs. [1–5]).

2. Iron overload in β-thalassemia

In β-thalassemia, as well as in other acquired and hereditary hemolytic anemia, iron overload is a common and serious complication and represents a major cause of morbidity and premature mortality in these patients. Hemoglobin instability, frequent blood transfusion, and increased iron absorption from the gastrointestinal tract represent the main causes of iron overload in β-thalassemia. Iron deposition occurs in visceral organs (mainly in the heart, liver, and endocrine glands), causing tissue damage and ultimately organ dysfunction and failure. Iron homeostasis depends on a coordinated regulation of molecules involved in the import of this element and those exporting it out of the cells. In particular, the iron status reflects the balance among iron uptake from the diet, its storage and mobilization, and its utilization [1]. Normally, 1–2 mg of iron is absorbed from the diet per day, with an equivalent amount lost by the turnover of gastrointestinal tract epithelial cells. In β-thalassemia and other transfusion-dependent anemias, iron overload may accumulate in relatively short time because there are no physiologically regulated means of iron excretion. Iron is essential for several vital biological processes. It regulates enzymatic activity and oxidation-reduction reactions playing a pivotal role in proliferation and cell survival. Iron ensures the transport of oxygen and the catalysis of reactions involved in electron transfer, DNA synthesis, and nitrogen fixation. However, it is also highly toxic due to its ability to react with oxygen and catalyze the production of reactive oxygen species (ROS). In solution, iron can exit in two states of oxidation, Fe (II) and Fe (III), and is very poorly soluble at physiological pH, especially when it is in the oxidized form Fe (III). Living organisms have thus developed many proteins to carry iron in biological fluids and transport it through cellular membranes and to store it in a non-toxic and easily mobilizable form [2, 6–8]. Iron is bound to transferrin in the plasma, but the iron overload in β-thalassemia patients saturates the ability of the transferrin iron transport system, leading to nontransferrin bound iron (NTBI) and labile plasma iron (LPI) starting to circulate in plasma and subsequently becoming deposited inside the susceptible cells [9, 10]. Rather than using the transferrin receptor, NTBI enters cells by nontransferrin pathways [1, 11]. Long-term uptake and accumulation of NTBI and LIP, its redox active component, lead to increate levels of storage iron and labile cellular iron [12]. Tissues susceptible to iron accumulation by this mechanism include the liver, endocrine system, and myocardium [13]. When the magnitude of the cellular LIP exceeds the capacity of the cell to synthesize new ferritin molecule, a critical concentration is reached that can generate reactive oxygen species (ROS). ROS produced by the metabolism of NTBI play a central role in inducing cellular dysfunction, apoptosis, and necrosis [14]. A variety of ROS, most notably hydroxyl radicals, increase lipid peroxidation and organelle damage, leading to cell death and fibrogenesis mediated by transforming growth factor β-1 (TGF-beta-1) [15]. An underappreciated effect of iron overload is increased the infection risk that is a high cause of mortality in β-thalassemia patients [16]. The LIP has been suggested as a low-molecular-weight intermediate or transitory pool between extracellular iron and intracellular firmly bound iron [17]. The intracellular LIP is redox active, catalyzing the Fenton and Haber-Weiss reactions that generate ROS [18]. Excess ROS are cytotoxic through their interaction with cellular components, such as DNA, proteins, and lipids, causing damage to vital organs [19].

3. Strategies to remove iron in excess

β-thalassemia is a significant health problem in various areas of the world due to its frequency and severity. The standard treatment of β-thalassemia is currently based on transfusion therapy, iron chelation, and, in rare cases, splenectomy. This has led to an increased survival and amelioration of the quality of life, although many patients continue to be affected by cardiac disease and other clinical complications, e.g., developed endocrine failure and delayed pubertal maturation. The only approach that may lead to a definitive cure for β-thalassemia is represented by allogenic hemopoietic stem cell transplantation, but the need to control transplant-related complications and the requirement for matched donors make this option not available to most patients. Thus, the main therapeutic option for the majority of patients remains to be supportive care in the form of blood transfusion combined with chelation therapy [2]. The function of iron chelators is that to remove excess iron from the plasma and the cells by binding the labile and chelatable iron, thus facilitating its excretion through the urine and feces. Deferoxamine was the first iron chelator to be used clinically and is given by a slow, continuous, subcutaneous, overnight infusion through a portable pump. Its side effects are minimal, but its mode of administration results in low compliance [1]. Deferasirox presents several side effects [1, 2]. Neutropenia is the main potential complication of deferiprone, the first effective oral iron chelator in removing excess iron from the organs and from the heart. The use of a combination of chelators leads to an improvement in the efficacy of chelation therapy: deferiprone may mobilize iron from tissues into the circulation, while deferoxamine binds and facilitates its excretion in the urine (the "shuttle mechanism") [1]. An additional potential approach to reduce iron overload is the downregulation of transferrin receptor 1 (TfR1) by administration of exogenous iron-free (apo) transferrin. In addition to free iron, some iron-containing compounds, due to hemolysis, are elevated in the plasma of β-thalassemia patients. They are free hemin and hemoglobin and are of considerable toxicity [1, 2]. These compounds are neutralized by their scavengers: hemopexin for free hemin and haptoglobin for free hemoglobin. These proteins are reduced in β-thalassemia patients, leaving free, un-neutralized hemin, and hemoglobin. The administration of hemopexin and haptoglobin may be suggested to reduce iron toxicity.

4. Strategies to modulate iron absorption

The discovery of hepcidin has led to an important advancement in the understanding of iron metabolism. Hepcidin is a key regulator of whole body iron homeostasis originally identified from urine as an antimicrobial peptide produced in the hepatocytes [20]. Mutations in the human HAMP gene or targeted deletion of the

HAMP gene in mice result in massive iron overload [21]. Conversely, high levels of hepcidin lead to decreased iron absorption and iron-restricted anemias indicating that hepcidin is a negative regulator of iron transport into plasma. Many experimental data suggested that the hepcidin could be the regulator of iron absorption and recycling acting principally or solely by binding to ferroportin, the only known cellular iron exporter. The systemic iron homeostasis is controlled by hepcidin-ferroportin interaction: hepcidin binds to ferroportin and induces its internalization and degradation, thus regulating the distribution of iron in the body. When hepcidin concentration increases, hepcidin binds to ferroportin, causing its phosphorylation, internalization, ubiquitylation, sorting through the multivesicular body pathway, and degradation in lysosomes, and iron is retained within the cells in cytoplasmic ferritin [22–25]. The expression of hepcidin is regulated by different stimuli at the transcriptional level: hypoxia, iron deficiency, erythroid expansion, and anemia are all negative regulators of hepcidin expression, while transferrin receptor 2 (TfR2), the membrane isoform of hemojuvelin (HJV), IL-6, iron, and the hemochromatosis protein HFE are all positive regulators of hepcidin transcription [2]. In β-thalassemia, in spite of iron overload, hepcidin production is generally low, and consequently, iron absorption is high. The process of differentiation and maturation of erythroid precursors is markedly altered in β-thalassemia (ineffective erythropoiesis). An excess of free α-globin chains within the red blood cells is the consequence of the reduced or lack synthesis of β-globin chains. Aggregation, denaturation, and degradation of these chains lead to the formation of insoluble precipitates that cause oxidative membrane damage within the red blood cell and developing erythroblasts (**Figure 1A**) [26]. Ineffective erythropoiesis is accompanied by a massive iron overload, due to an increase in iron absorption by the gastrointestinal tract and to frequent blood transfusions. Nevertheless, iron overload occurs also in patients who have not received transfusions such as patients suffering from thalassemia intermedia [27, 28]. If iron was a dominant regulator, patients with β-thalassemia should express very high levels of hepcidin in serum in order to decrease intestinal iron absorption. By contrast, the levels of hepcidin are very low in these patients, suggesting that the ineffective erythropoiesis alone is able to suppress the synthesis of hepcidin in spite of the presence of a severe iron overload [25, 29–31]. Transfusions of erythrocyte partially rerelieved suppression of hepcidin, but transfusions add large amounts of exogenous iron and lead to iron overload. Hepcidin mRNA expression in the HepG2 cell line by serum from β-thalassemia patients suggested the existence of a negative erythropoietic regulator of hepcidin expression [32]. The nature of this humoral factor is still uncharacterized but may include growth differentiation factor (GDF-15), twisted gastrulation protein homolog 1 (TWSG1), soluble transferrin receptor, and erythroferrone, which are all overproduced by the proliferating erythroid precursors (**Figure 2**). Controlling absorption of iron may be beneficial to the administration of synthetic hepcidin or of agents that increase its expression. Hepcidin agonists or stimulators of hepcidin production are being developed for the treatment or prevention of iron overload in hepcidin deficiency states, including hereditary hemochromatosis and β-thalassemia [33]. The rationale for the use of hepcidin agonists is justified by two principal observations: first, the phlebotomy is an expensive and effective treatment for iron overload that is acceptable to must but not all patients affected by hereditary hemochromatosis; second, iron-loading anemias cannot be treated in this way and require iron chelation therapy, which is not well tolerate by many patients. Hepcidin agonists are agents that replace hepcidin activity or stimulate its endogenous production and, in both hereditary hemochromatosis and iron loading anemia, could prevent iron accumulation by redistributing iron from parenchymal tissues to macrophages where iron is less toxic [34, 35].

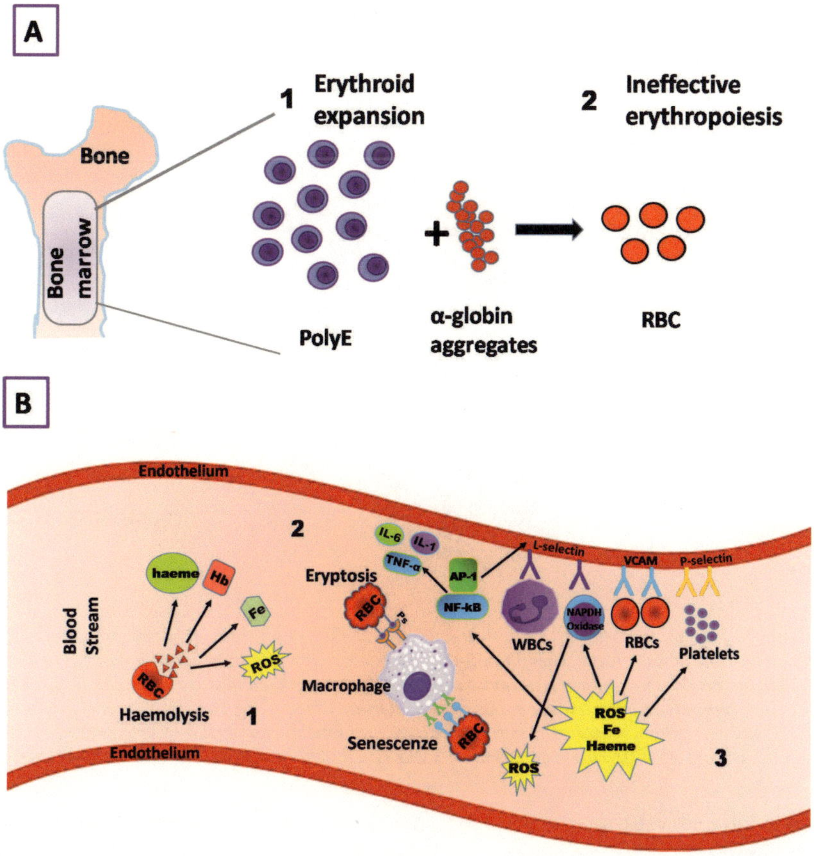

Figure 1.
(A) Erythroid expansion and ineffective erythropoiesis represent oxidative events in the bone marrow. (B). Oxidative events in the circulation: (1) hemolysis leads to hemoglobin release in the plasma. Autoxidation of free hemoglobin produces ROS, free heme, and iron; (2) eryptosis and senescence: two different mechanisms of endocytosis of red blood cells (RBCs) by macrophages; and (3) membrane oxidative damage by ROS, free heme, and iron: activation of NF-κB and AP-1 by ROS and heme increases the production of pro-inflammatory cytokines (IL-1, IL-6, and TNFα) and adhesion molecules on the endothelium. Activated leucocytes generate more ROS by their NAPDH oxidase, creating a loop of oxidative stress and inflammation.

TMPRSS6 suppression could be an alternative approach to increase hepatic synthesis of hepcidin. It is a transmembrane serine protease (matriptase-2) that normally suppresses the synthesis of hepcidin by deactivating hemojuvelin (HJV) [36]. Data showed that the deletion of TMPRSS6 gene in mouse model increased hepcidin expression resulting in anemia improvement, ineffective erythropoiesis, and splenomegaly reducing and decreased iron loading [37]. An improvement in anemia and iron overload has been showed in mice and in preclinical studies using antisense oligonucleotides or small interfering RNAs (siRNA9 decreasing TMPRSS6) [38, 39]. The somministration of exogenous transferrin, through the downregulation of TfR1, increased erythroid precursor enucleation and improved terminal erythroid differentiation and maturation in β-thalassemic mice [40, 41]. Recently, a new iron metabolism regulating factor produced in erythroblasts in response to erythropoietin, ERFE (erythroferrone), was identified. In murine models with β-thalassemia intermedia, ERFE is highly expressed and mediates hepcidin suppression and contributes to iron overload. On the contrary, a deficiency of ERFE leads to an increase in hepcidin expression, a significant reduction in iron overload, and a slight improvement of erythropoietic indices [42]. All these data indicate that the inhibition of ERFE may be a future target with therapeutic potential in diseases

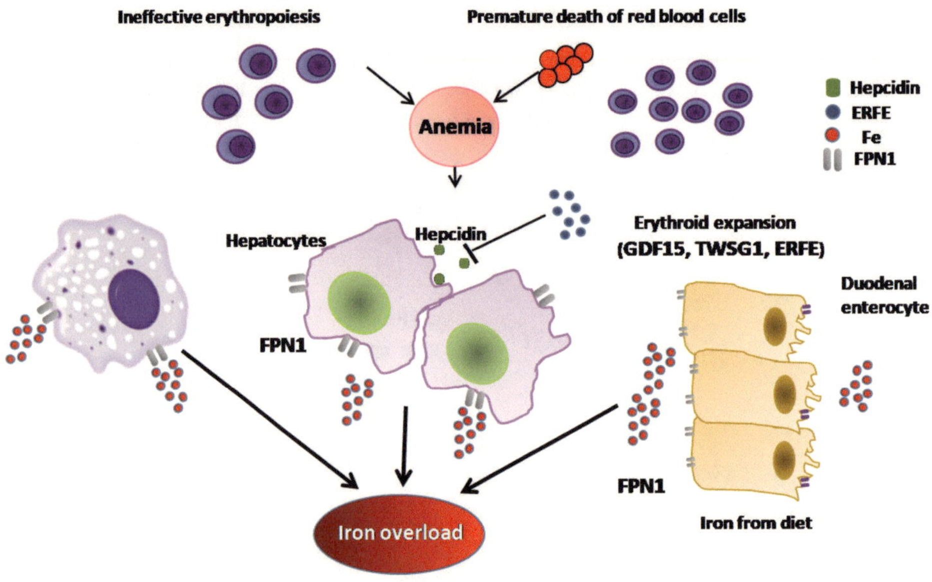

Figure 2.
Dysregulation of iron homeostasis in β-thalassemia disease. Ineffective erythropoiesis and premature death of red blood cells are the main cause of anemia in β-thalassemia patients. Erythropoietin production induced by anemia causes an increase in erythropoiesis activating secretion of erythroid factors such as GDF15, TWSG1, and ERFE. The suppression of hepcidin expression caused by an excess of eryhtroid factors leads to an increase in intestinal iron absorption, release of iron from the liver, and reticuloendothelial system. All these lead to iron overload. GDF15: Growth differentiation factor 15; TWSG1: Twisted-gastrulation 1; ERFE: Erythroferrone.

with ineffective erythropoiesis and iron overload as β-thalassemia. Agents targeting hepcidin expression are more likely to be beneficial to patients with NTDT than those with TDT because transfusional iron overload is not mediated by low hepcidin levels. However, mini-hepcidins and TMRSS6 inhibitors can be evaluated for use in patients with TDT because improvement in erythropoiesis could potentially reduce transfusion requirements [43]. All discussed novel agents merit further evaluation of efficacy and safety in both preclinical and clinical development studies.

5. Oxidative stress in β-thalassemia

Oxidative stress plays a major role in pathophysiology of β-thalassemia, although it is not the primary etiology of disease. The cell oxidative status depends on the equilibrium between oxidants and anti-oxidants. The reactive oxygen species (ROS) are oxidants produced mainly as byproducts of cellular respiration, while reduced glutathione is an example of anti-oxidants. A balance between oxidants and anti-oxidants is crucial for normal physiology. ROS are utilized from the cells as regulators in many physiological processes, including proliferation and differentiation of the erythroid precursors. Oxidative stress ensues in many pathological processes when the balance between oxidants and anti-oxidants is broken, as it occurs in β-thalassemia. Excess ROS cause cytotoxicity by binding to cell components such as DNA, proteins, and membrane lipids [19]. In β-thalassemia, the main consequence of the unstable Hb_s and iron overload is the oxidative stress. It mediates many of symptoms due to oxidative damage to red blood cells, leukocytes (recurrent infections), platelets (hypercoagulable state), as well as in heart, liver, and the endocrine glands (**Figures 1A** and **B**) [19, 44–46]. Endogenous and exogenous antioxidants may ameliorate the oxidative stress in β-thalassemia. They act scavenging and inactivating ROS and correcting their damage to cellular components. We introduce many antioxidants by nutrition. For example, a moderate wine consumption and a "Mediterranean diet" are thought to have a protective effect due to their high contents of antioxidants [47, 48]. Antioxidants can also be taken as food additives, or as crude extracts, such as preparation of papaya fermented and curcumin, either as pure compounds such as vitamins C and E and Q10 [49]. An improvement in many parameters of oxidative stress by using such additives in β-thalassemia was observed, but a clear clinical benefit, such as reducing transfusion dependence, was less successful. A combination of drugs affecting both the oxidative stress and the iron overload can give an effective outcome. Forkhead-box-O3 (Foxo3) is a critical transcription factor that protects the cell from oxidative stress by upregulating antioxidant enzymes during early stages of erythropoiesis [50]. At early stages, Foxo3 is phosphorylated by proteins of the EPOR-P13K/AKT/mTOR signaling pathway and is translocated out of the nucleus, where it remains inactivated. At late stages, Foxo3 is relocated into the nucleus, gets activated, and induces the production of antioxidants that neutralize ROS to allow efficient erythropoiesis [1, 36, 51, 52]. In mice with β-thalassemia intermedia, downregulation of Foxo3, as a result of persistent activation of EPOR-p13K/AKT/mTOR pathway, was observed. Inactivation of Foxo3 leads to oxidative damage in late erythroblasts and plays a significant role in the process of ineffective erythropoiesis [53]. β-thalassemia patients could be beneficial in improving anemia by activation of Foxo3 as a potential inducer of HbF. However, the function of Foxo3 in hemoglobinopathies has yet to be elucidated. A remarkable improvement in erythroid cell maturation, production of β-globin chains, and anemia has been observed following the use of rapamycin, an mTOR inhibition, in mice with β-thalassemia intermedia [53]. In another study, rapamycin increased α-globin expression and HbF production in cultured erythroid precursors from patients with β-thalassemia intermedia [54, 55]. Similar findings were reported with the use of another Foxo3 activating agent, resveratrol (3,5,4′-trihydroxy-trans-stilbene), a non-flavonoid polyphenol that upregulates antioxidant enzymes in mice with β-thalassemia intermedia [56]. Metformin, an approved drug for diabetes type 2 and a Foxo3 inducer, has been investigated as an HbF inducer in an ongoing phase 1 clinical trial in patients with sickle cell anemia and nontransfusion-dependent thalassemia (NTDT; NCT02981329) [57]. All these agents are in preclinical studies and need further evaluation. Then, further laboratory and clinical investigations are required in this field. A factor required for the initiation of translation through the binding of tRNA to the ribosomes is the eukaryotic initiation factor 2 (eIF2). It is regulated by a mechanism involving phosphorylation at its α-subunit by heme-regulated eIF2a kinase (HRI) in the erythroid precursors. Stress, as heme deficiency and oxidative stress during the late stage of erythroid differentiation, activates HRI that coordinates the synthesis of heme and globin. It was demonstrated that the phosphorylated α-subunit of eIF2 turned on the activating transcription factor 4 (ATF4) to diminish oxidative stress in erythroid precursors [58–60]. A selective inhibitor of eIF2aP dephosphorylation as salubrinal augmented the HRI signaling pathway and reduced the production of hemichromes in β-thalassemia erythroid precursors [59]. In another study, salubrinal increased HbF production with a concomitant decrease of HbA in differentiating human CD34 cells by a post-transcriptional mechanism [61]. Thus, manipulation of the HRI-eIF2aP signaling pathway could represent a new approach for the treatment of β-thalassemia.

An antioxidant protein that scavenges and inactivates ROS is the peroxiredoxin-2 (Prx2), essential during erythropoiesis. The expression of this protein is upregulated both murine and human β-thalassemia indicating that the oxidative stress induces peroxiredoxin-2 as a novel cytoprotective response in β-thalassemic erythropoiesis [62, 63]. Heme oxygenase (HO-1) is an enzyme that catalyzes the degradation of heme in response to stress, such as oxidative stress or hypoxia, both of which occur in β-thalassemia. In EPO-dependent fetal liver erythropoietic cells from β-thalassemic mice, the expression of HO-1 was augmented. The administration of tin protoporphyrin IX, an HO-1 inhibitor, improved ineffective erythropoiesis and Hb levels and decreased spleen size and liver iron [64, 65].

6. Potential role of antioxidants in β-thalassemia

Various antioxidant enzyme systems are activated by the oxidative stress to protect the body tissues from its damaging effects in β-thalassemia patients. These antioxidants include superoxide dismutase (SOD), catalase, glutathione (GSH), thioredoxin (Trx), and ferritin. Superoxide (O_2^-) is the first reactive radical produced, and this radical can be neutralized by SOD. There are three distinct SODs: SOD1 (cu/Zn-SOD) is present in cytoplasm, whereas SOD2 (Mn-SOD) is present in the mitochondria, and SOD3 is almost exclusively extracellular [66, 67]. Each of these distinct SODs performs a specific function in human cells. In β-thalassemia, major patients higher levels of erythrocyte superoxide dismutase and glutathione peroxidase (GPx) as well as higher plasma malondialdehyde (MDA) were observed as compared to healthy controls [68]. Iron overload through repeated blood transfusions and subsequent oxidative stress produced by reactive oxygen species may be the cause of increased levels of MDA. The rise in SOD and glutathione peroxidase may occur as a result of compensatory mechanisms in response to oxidative stress [44]. Neutralization of O_2^- produces H_2O_2, which can be metabolized into nontoxic products by a catalase and glutathione peroxidase (GPx) in conjunction with glutathione. Location of GPx depends on the subtype, whereas catalase is present in peroxisomes [67]. The stability of the cellular and subcellular membranes depends mainly on glutathione peroxidase, and the protective antioxidant effect of glutathione peroxidase depends on the presence of selenium. In patients with β-thalassemia, major was confirmed the peroxidative status generated by iron overload and the high increase in serum ferritin, iron, plasmatic thiobarbituric acid reactive substances (TBARS), SOD, and glutathione peroxidase activity, while the vitamin E and zinc concentration decreased in these patients [44, 69]. Glutathione (GSH) is present in nearly all cells in the body and is present in high levels in organs with high oxygen consumption and energy production, e.g., the brain [67, 70]. Glutathione, in conjunction with its oxidized form (GSSG), plays a major role in controlling cellular redox state. The ubiquitous thioredoxin system also plays an important role in maintaining the cell's redox state [67, 71]. Finally, ferritin is considered an endogenous antioxidant as it performs the important function of sequestering potentially toxic labile iron. When endogenous antioxidants are unable to neutralize oxidative stress, as in β-thalassemia, exogenous antioxidants can be used to augment the antioxidant system of the body. Iron metabolism underlies the dynamic interplay between oxidative stress and antioxidants in many pathophysiological processes. Iron overload can affect redox state, and not only this condition can be restored to physiological conditions using iron chelation, but also the addition of antioxidants to these treatment regimens can be a viable therapeutic approach for attenuating tissue damage induced by oxidative stress (**Table 1**), (**Figure 3**, [72–74]). Vitamin A (β-carotene), vitamin C, vitamin E (α-tocopherol), polyphenols, and other bioactive plant-derived compounds are effective exogenous antioxidants that also regulate iron metabolism. At the transcriptional level, antioxidant enzymes are regulated by the transcription factor Nrf2, which binds to the antioxidant response element (ARE) in the target gene's promoter region. Nrf2 is believed to be phosphorylated by protein kinase C (PKC), which causes the transcription factor to translocate to the nucleus, where it activates ARE-containing genes [67, 75], ultimately leading

Antioxidant	Mechanisms of iron regulation	Sources of antioxidants
Curcumin	• Potent flavonoid antioxidant • Iron chelator • Redox state modulator • Decreased iron levels • Attenuated lipopolysaccharide (LPS)-induced oxidative stress-related inflammation • Activated hepatic IRPs and TfR1, repressed hepatic hepcidin and ferritin synthesis	Curcumin is a bright yellow chemical produced by *Curcuma longa* plants
Quercetin	• Decreased hepatic iron levels • Reduced iron-related damage • Increased BMP6, intranuclear SMAD4, SMAD4 binding to the HAMP promoter, and hepcidin expression	Vegetables, leaves, grains, red onions, kale, red wine, and tea
Flavonoid-rich extract of orange and bergamot juice	• Decreased ROS production and membrane lipid peroxidation by iron chelation in iron-overload A549 cells and activation of antioxidant catalase enzyme	Citrus fruits
Genistein	• Reduced inflammation induced by ethanol and oxidative stress in mice • Increased HAMP promoter activity in both zebrafish and human hepatocytes via Stat3- and Smad4-dependent process	Lupin, fava beans, soy beans, kudzu, psoralea, *Maackia amurensis*, and *Flemingia vestita*
Silymarine	• Iron-chelating properties	*Silybum marianum* extract
Ferulic acid	• Decreased iron-induced oxidative stress, reduced liver injury, and ROS production • Increased hepatic antioxidant and mitochondrial membrane potential	Vegetables, popcorn, bamboo shoots, cereals (bran, wheat, and barley grain)
Resveratrol	• Reduced myocardial damage by modulating vascular cell function, low density lipoprotein (LDL) oxidation, and platelet aggregation	Skin of grapes, blueberries, raspberries, mulberries, peanuts, and red wine

Table 1.
Mechanisms of iron regulation by antioxidants.

to the neutralization of free radicals and the attenuation of oxidative damage [76]. **Table 1** summarizes the flavonoids and other antioxidants that regulate both iron homeostasis and redox state, in some cases via independent mechanisms. Flavonoids are present in a wide variety of plants and represent the most common class of polyphenols, organic chemicals that protect the plant from ultraviolet radiation, pathogens, and effects of oxidative stress, making them suitable for therapeutic purposes [77, 78]. Examples of flavonoids include quercetin, cathechins, curcumin, and kaempferol, which are abundant in fruits, vegetables, legumes, red wine, and green tea. Curcumin is a potent flavonoid antioxidant that can chelate iron in addition to modulating redox state [79]. A flavonoid-rich extract of orange and bergamot juice has been shown to chelate iron in iron-overload A549 cells and to activate the antioxidant enzyme catalase, leading to a decrease in ROS production and membrane lipid peroxidation [80]. It is a promising candidate for regulating both oxidative stress and iron homeostasis. Quercetin can reduce hepatic iron deposition in mice

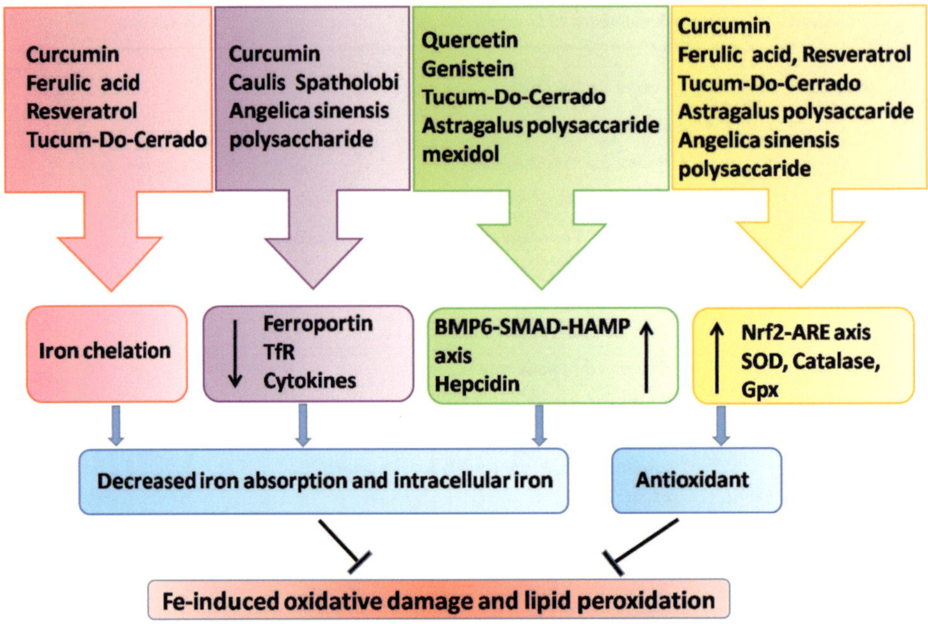

Figure 3.
Summary of the mechanisms regulating iron and oxidative stress by antioxidants. BMP6-SMAD-HAMP: Bone morphogenetic factor-mothers against decapentaplegic homolog-hepcidin antimicrobial peptide; GPx: Glutathione peroxidase;Nrf2-ARE: Nuclear factor erythroid 2-related factor 2-antioxidant response element; SOD: Superoxide dismutase.

that were exposed to either ethanol or excess iron and increase BMP6, intranuclear SMAD4, SMAD4 binding to the HAMP promoter, and hepcidin expression, leading to decreased hepatic iron levels and reduced iron-related damage [81]. Another potent antioxidant is genistein. It reduces inflammation induced by ethanol and oxidative stress in mice [82] and, similar to quercetin, increases HAMP promoter activity in both zebrafish and human hepatocytes via Stat3- and Smad4-dependent process [83]. Silymarin, another flavonoid, is present in milk thistle plant extract and may have iron-chelating properties [84]. It is safe, well tolerated, cost-effective alternative to currently available iron chelation therapies for treating patients with β-thalassemia [84]. Ferulic acid is present in a wide variety of plants, and the antioxidant effects are believed to be mediated via the neutralization of free radicals [85]. The antioxidant effects of resveratrol may prevent adverse changes that lead to cardiovascular disease by modulating vascular cell function, low density lipoprotein (LDL) oxidation, and platelet aggregation, thereby reducing myocardial damage [86, 87]. Both vitamin A and vitamin C have well-established antioxidant properties that are mediated via the attenuation of oxidative damage [88]. Vitamin A and β-carotene increase hepcidin and TfR expression and intestinal iron absorption, reduce inflammatory signaling and ferroportin expression, increase intracellular ferritin levels, and release intracellular trapped iron [89–91]. Vitamin C reduces Fe^{3+} to Fe^{2+} and inhibits hepcidin expression [92]. In recent years, research for new therapies based on plant-derived compounds has developed considerably. This is to maximize the benefits of plant phytochemicals and avoid the adverse effects often associated with synthetic pharmaceutical agents [93]. Several plant extracts, such as tucum-do-cerrado, astragalus, *Angelica sinensis*, *Caulis Spatholobi*, *Scutellaria baicalensis*, and others, have been studied for their putative effects on iron homeostasis and oxidative stress. The results obtained are very promising (for esaustive review, see Ref. [76]).

7. Conclusions

Alteration in iron homeostasis is associated with oxidative stress and inflammation. Many bioactive antioxidants and plant-derived phytochemicals can regulate iron homeostasis, inflammation, and oxidative stress. Nevertheless, the majority of data collected to date are derived from in vitro and animal experiments, and further studies are needed in order to evaluate the efficacy of these phytochemicals as a natural substitute for pharmaceutical agents. This is very important because many pharmaceutical agents are associated with adverse side effects.

Author details

Nadia Maria Sposi
Center for Gender-Specific Medicine, Istituto Superiore di Sanità, Rome, Italy

*Address all correspondence to: nadia.sposi@iss.it

References

[1] Fibach E, Rachmilewitz EA. Pathophysiology and treatment of patients with beta-thalassemia - an update. F1000Res. 2017;**6**:2156. DOI: 10.12688/f1000research.12688.1

[2] Sposi NM. In: Munshi A, editor. Interaction between Erythropoiesis and Iron Metabolism in Human β-Thalassemia - Recent Advances and New Therapeutic Approaches, Inherited Hemoglobin Disorders. Rijeka: IntechOpen; 2015. DOI: 10.5772/61716

[3] Galanello R, Origa R. Beta-thalassemia. Orphanet Journal of Rare Diseases. 2010;**21**:5-11. DOI: 10.1186/1750-1172-5-11

[4] Weatherall DJ, Clegg JB, Higgs DR, Wood WG. The hemoglobinopathies. In: Scriver CR, Beaudet AL, Sly WS, Valle D, Vogelstein B, editors. The Metabolic and Molecular Bases of Inherited Disease (OMMBID); Chapter 101. New York, NY: McGraw-Hill; 2002

[5] Cao A, Galanello R. Beta-thalassemia. Genetics in Medicine. 2010;**12**(2):61-76

[6] Beaumont C, Vaulont S. Iron homeostasis. Iron homeostasis. In: ESH Handbook on Disorders of Iron Metabolism. Chapter 20. 2009. pp. 488-511

[7] Hentze MW, Muckenthaler MV, Andrews NC. Balancing acts: Molecular control of mammalian iron metabolism. Cell. 2004;**117**:285-297

[8] Yun S, Vincelette ND. Update on iron metabolism and molecular perspective of common genetic and acquired disorder, hemochromatosis. Critical Reviews in Oncology/Hematology. 2015;**95**(1):12-25. DOI: 10.1016/j.critrevonc

[9] Leecharoenkiat K, Lithanatudom P, Sornjai W, Smith DR. Iron dysregulation in beta-thalassemia. Asian Pacific Journal of Tropical Medicine. 2016;**9**(11):1035-1043. DOI: 10.1016/j.apjtm.2016.07.035

[10] Hershko C. Pathogenesis and management of iron toxicity in thalassemia. Annals of the New York Academy of Sciences. 2010:1-9

[11] Prus E, Fibach E. Uptake of non-transferrin iron by erythroid cells. Anemia. 2011;**2011**:945289. DOI: 10.1155/2011/945289

[12] Cabantchik ZI. Labile iron in cells and body fluids: Physiology, pathology, and pharmacology. Frontiers in Pharmacology. 2014;**5**:45

[13] Murphy CJ, Oudit GY. Iron-overload cardiomyopathy: Pathophysiology, diagnosis, and treatment. Journal of Cardiac Failure. 2010;**16**(11):888-900

[14] Bresgen N, Eckl PM. Oxidative stress and the homeodynamics of iron metabolism. Biomolecules. 2015;**5**(2):808-847

[15] Jain M, Rivera S, Monclus EA, Synenki L, Zirk A, Eisenbart J, et al. Mitochondrial reactive oxygen species regulate transforming growth factor-beta signaling. Journal of Biological Chemistry. 2013;**288**(2):770-777

[16] Telfer PT, Warburton F, Christou S, Hadjigavriel M, Sitarou M, Kolnagou A, et al. Improved survival in thalassemia major patients on switching from desferrioxamine to combined chelation therapy with desferrioxamine and deferiprone. Haematologica. 2009;**94**(12):1777-1778

[17] Jacobs A. Low molecular weight intracellular iron transport compounds. Blood. 1977;**50**(3):433-439

[18] Jacobs A. An intracellular transit iron pool. CIBA Foundation Symposium. 1976;**51**:91-106

[19] Fibach E, Rachmilewitz E. The role of oxidative stress in hemolytic anemia. Current Molecular Medicine. 2008;**8**(7):609-619

[20] Park CH, Valore EV, Waring AJ, Ganz T. Hepcidin, a urinary antimicrobial peptide synthesized in the liver. Journal of Biological Chemistry. 2001;**276**:7806-7810

[21] Nicolas G, Bennoun M, Devaux I, Beaumont C, Grandchamp B, Kahn A, et al. Lack of hepcidin gene expression and severe tissue iron overload in upstream stimulatory factor 2 (USF2) knockout mice. Proceedings of the National Academy of Sciences of the United States of America. 2001;**98**:8780-8785

[22] Cianetti L, Gabbianelli M, Sposi NM. Ferroportin and erythroid cells: an update. Advances in Hematology. 2010;**2010**:404173

[23] Evstatiev R, Gasche C. Iron sensing and signaling. Gut. 2012;**61**:933-952

[24] Fleming RE, Sly WS. Hepcidin: A putative iron regulatory hormone relevant to hereditary hemochromatosis and the anemia of chronic disease. Proceedings of the National Academy of Sciences of the United States of America. 2001;**98**:8160-8162

[25] Piperno A, Mariani R, Trombini P, Girelli D. Hepcidin modulation in human diseases: From research to clinic. World Journal of Gastroenterology. 2009;**15**:538-551

[26] Melchiori L, Gardenghi S, Rivella S. Beta-Thalassemia: HiJAKing Ineffective Erythropoiesis and Iron Overload. Advances in Hematology. 2010;**2010**:938640. DOI: 10.1155/2010/938640

[27] Ribeil JA, Arlet JB, Dussiot M, Moura IC, Courtois G, Hermine O. Ineffective erythropoiesis in β-thalassemia. Hindawi Publishing Corporation. The Scientific World Journal. 2013;**2013**:394295

[28] Visvader JE, Mao X, Fujiwara Y, Hahm K, Orkin SH. The LIM-domain binding protein Ldb1 and its partner LMO2 act as negative regulators of erythroid differentiation. Proceedings of the National Academy of Sciences of the United States of America. 1997;**94**(25):13707-13712

[29] Ganz T. Hepcidin, a key regulator of iron metabolism and mediator of anemia of inflammation. Blood. 2003;**102**:783-788

[30] Papanikolaou G, Tzilianos JI, Christakis JI, Bogdanos D, Tsimirika K, MacFarlane J, et al. Hepcidin in iron overload disorders. Blood. 2005;**105**:4103-4105

[31] Kattamis A, Papassotiriou I, Palaiologou D, Apostolakou F, Galani A, Ladis V, et al. The effects of erythropoietic activity and iron burden on hepcidin expression in patients with thalassemia major. Haematologica. 2006;**91**:809-812

[32] Weizer-Stern O, Adamsky K, Amariglio N, Levin C, Koren A, Breuer W, et al. Downregulation of hepcidin and haemojuvelin expression in the hepatocyte cell-line HepG2 induced by thalassemic sera. British Journal of Haematology. 2006;**135**:129-138

[33] Ganz T. Hepcidin and iron regulation, 10 years later. Blood. 2011;**117**:4425-4433

[34] Ganz T, Nemeth E. The hepcidin-ferroportin system as a therapeutic target in anemias and iron overload. Hematology. American Society of Hematology. Education Program. 2011;**2011**:538-542

[35] Gardenghi S, Ramos P, Marongiu MF, Melchiori L, Breda L, Guy E, et al. Hepcidin as a therapeutic tool to limit iron overload and improve anemia in β-thalassemic mice. The Journal of Clinical Investigation. 2010;**120**:4466-4477

[36] El-Beshlawy A, El-Ghamrawy M. Recent trends in treatment of thalassemia. Blood Cells, Molecules & Diseases. 2019;**76**:53-58

[37] Nai A, Pagani A, Mandelli G, Lidonnici MR, Silvestri L, Ferrari G, et al. Deletion of TMPRSS6 attenuates the phenotype in a mouse model of β-thalassemia. Blood. 2012;**119**(21):5021-5029. DOI: 10.1182/blood-2012-01-401885

[38] Guo S, Casu C, Gardenghi S, Booten S, Aghajan M, Peralta R, et al. Reducing TMPRSS6 ameliorates hemochromatosis and β-thalassemia in mice. The Journal of Clinical Investigation. 2013;**123**(4):1531-1541. DOI: 10.1172/JCI66969

[39] Schmidt PJ, Toudjarska I, Sendamarai AK, Racie T, Milstein S, Bettencourt BR, et al. An RNAi therapeutic targeting Tmprss6 decreases iron overload in Hfe(-/-) mice and ameliorates anemia and iron overload in murine β-thalassemia intermedia. Blood. 2013;**121**(7):1200-1208. DOI: 10.1182/blood-2012-09-453977

[40] Li H, Rybicki AC, Suzuka SM, von Bonsdorff L, Breuer W, Hall CB, et al. Transferrin therapy ameliorates disease in beta-thalassemic mice. Nature Medicine. 2010;**16**(2):177-182. DOI: 10.1038/nm.2073

[41] Li H, Choesang T, Bao W, Chen H, Feola M, Garcia-Santos D, et al. Decreasing TfR1 expression reverses anemia and hepcidin suppression in β-thalassemic mice. Blood. 2017;**129**(11):1514-1526. DOI: 10.1182/blood-2016-09-742387

[42] Kautz L, Jung G, Du X, Gabayan V, Chapman J, Nasoff M, et al. Erythroferrone contributes to hepcidin suppression and iron overload in a mouse model of β-thalassemia. Blood. 2015;**126**(17):2031-2037. DOI: 10.1182/blood-2015-07-658419

[43] Cappellini MD, Porter JB, Viprakasit V, Taher AT. A paradigm shift on beta-thalassaemia treatment: How will we manage this old disease with new therapies? Blood Reviews. 2018;**32**(4):300-311. DOI: 10.1016/j.blre.2018.02.001

[44] Shazia Q, Mohammad ZH, Rahman T, Shekhar HU. Correlation of oxidative stress with serum trace element levels and antioxidant enzyme status in Beta- thalassemia major patients: A review of the literature. Anemia. 2012;**2012**:270923. DOI: 10.1155/2012/270923

[45] Pavlova LE, Savov VM, Petkov HG, Charova IP. Oxidative stress in patients with beta-thalassemia major. Prilozi. 2007;**28**(1):145-154

[46] Ghone RA, Kumbar KM, Suryakar AN, Katkam RV, Joshi NG. Oxidative stress and disturbance in antioxidant balance in beta thalassemia major. Indian Journal of Clinical Biochemistry. 2008;**23**(4):337-340

[47] Khemayanto H, Shi B. Role of Mediterranean diet in prevention and management of type 2 diabetes. Chinese Medical Journal. 2014;**127**(20):3651-3656

[48] Hu X, Wang H, Lv X, Chu L, Liu Z, Wei X, et al. Cardioprotective effects of tannic acid on isoproterenol-induced myocardial injury in rats: Further insight into 'French paradox'. Phytotherapy Research. 2015;**29**(9):1295-1303

[49] Fibach E, Rachmilewitz EA. The role of antioxidants and iron chelators

in the treatment of oxidative stress in thalassemia. Annals of the New York Academy of Sciences. 2010;**1202**:10-6. DOI: 10.1111/j.1749-6632.2010.05577.x

[50] Liang R, Ghaffari S. Advances in understanding the mechanisms of erythropoiesis in homeostasis and disease. British Journal of Haematology. 2016;**174**(5):661-673

[51] Marinkovic D, Zhang X, Yalcin S, Luciano JP, Brugnara C, Huber T, et al. Foxo3 is required for the regulation of oxidative stress in erythropoiesis. The Journal of Clinical Investigation. 2007;**117**(8):2133-2144

[52] Wang H, Li Y, Wang S, Zhang Q, Zheng J, Yang Y, et al. Knockdown of transcription factor forkhead box O3 (FOXO3) suppresses erythroid differentiation in human cells and zebrafish. Biochemical and Biophysical Research Communications. 2015;**460**(4):923-930

[53] Zhang X, Campreciós G, Rimmelé P, Liang R, Yalcin S, Mungamuri SK, et al. FOXO3-mTOR metabolic cooperation in the regulation of erythroid cell maturation and homeostasis. American Journal of Hematology. 2014;**89**:954-963

[54] Pecoraro A, Troia A, Calzolari R, Scazzone C, Rigano P, Martorana A, et al. Efficacy of rapamycin as inducer of Hb F in primary Erythroid cultures from sickle cell disease and β-thalassemia patients. Hemoglobin. 2015;**39**(4):225-229

[55] Bianchi N, Zuccato C, Lampronti I, Borgatti M, Gambari R. Fetal hemoglobin inducers from the natural world: a novel approach for identification of drugs for the treatment of β-thalassemia and sickle-cell anemia. Evidence-based Complementary and Alternative Medicine. 2009;**6**(2):141-151. DOI: 10.1093/ecam/nem139

[56] Franco SS, De Falco L, Ghaffari S, Brugnara C, Sinclair DA, Matte' A, et al. Resveratrol accelerates erythroid maturation by activation of FoxO3 and ameliorates anemia in beta thalassemic mice. Haematologica. 2014;**99**:267-275

[57] Zhang Y, Weiss M, Sumazin P, Sheehan VA. Metformin induces FOXO3-dependent fetal hemoglobin production in primary erythroid cells [abstract]. Blood. 2016;**128**(22):321-333

[58] Donnelly N, Gorman AM, Gupta S, Samali A. The eIF2α kinases: Their structures and functions. Cellular and Molecular Life Sciences. 2013;**70**(19):3493-3511. DOI: 10.1007/s00018-012-1252-6

[59] Chen JJ. Translational control by heme-regulated eIF2α kinase during erythropoiesis. Current Opinion in Hematology. 2014;**21**(3):172-178

[60] Suragani RN, Zachariah RS, Velazquez JG, Liu S, Sun CW, Townes TM, et al. Heme-regulated eIF2α kinase activated Atf4 signaling pathway in oxidative stress and erythropoiesis. Blood. 2012;**119**(22):5276-5284. DOI: 10.1182/blood-2011-10-388132

[61] Hahn CK, Lowrey CH. Induction of fetal hemoglobin through enhanced translation efficiency of γ-globin mRNA. Blood. 2014;**124**(17):2730-2734. DOI: 10.1182/blood-2014-03-564302

[62] De Franceschi L, Bertoldi M, De Falco L, Santos Franco S, Ronzoni L, Turrini F, et al. Oxidative stress modulates heme synthesis and induces peroxiredoxin-2 as a novel cytoprotective response in β-thalassemic erythropoiesis. Haematologica. 2011;**96**(11):1595-1604. DOI: 10.3324/haematol.2011.043612

[63] Matte A, De Falco L, Iolascon A, Mohandas N, An X, Siciliano A, et al. The interplay between Peroxiredoxin-2 and nuclear factor-Erythroid 2 is

important in limiting oxidative mediated dysfunction in β-Thalassemic erythropoiesis. Antioxidants & Redox Signaling. 2015;**23**(16):1284-1297

[64] Pittalà V, Salerno L, Romeo G, Modica MN, Siracusa MA. A focus on heme oxygenase-1 (HO-1) inhibitors. Current Medicinal Chemistry. 2013;**20**(30):3711-3732

[65] Santos DG, Mikhael M, Rivella S, et al. Heme Oxygenase 1 plays a role In the pathophysiology of beta-thalassemia. Blood. 2015;**122**

[66] Hou W, Xie Y, Song X, Sun X, Lotze MT, Zeh HJ, et al. Autophagy promotes ferroptosis by degradation of ferritin. Autophagy. 2016;**12**:1425-1428. DOI: 10.1080/15548627.2016.1187366

[67] Crichton RR, Wilmet S, Legssyer R, Ward RJ. Molecular and cellular mechanisms of iron homeostasis and toxicity in mammalian cells. Journal of Inorganic Biochemistry. 2002;**91**:9-18. DOI: 10.1016/S0162-0134(02)00461-0

[68] Filiz S, Gulyuz O, Sabri K, Deniz E, Alev H. Oxidant and antioxidant status in beta thalassemia major patients. Journal of Ankara University Faculty of. Medicine. 2005;**58**(1):34-38

[69] Kassab-Chekir A, Laradi S, Ferchichi S, Haj Khelil A, Feki M, Amri F, et al. Oxidant, antioxidant status and metabolic data in patients with beta-thalassemia. Clinica Chimica Acta. 2003;**338**(1-2):79-86

[70] Zelko IN, Mariani TJ, Folz RJ. Superoxide dismutase multigene family: A comparison of the CuZn-SOD (SOD1), Mn-SOD (SOD2), and EC-SOD (SOD3) gene structures, evolution, and expression. Free Radical Biology & Medicine. 2002;**33**:337-349. DOI: 10.1016/S0891-5849(02)00905-X

[71] Wu G, Fang YZ, Yang S, Lupton JR, Turner ND. Glutathione metabolism and its implications for health. The Journal of Nutrition. 2004;**134**:489-492

[72] Grune T, Sommerburg O, Siems WG. Oxidative stress in anemia. Clinical Nephrology. 2000;**53**:S18-S22

[73] Temple NJ. Antioxidants and disease: More questions than answers. Nutrition Research. 2000;**20**:449-459. DOI: 10.1016/S0271-5317(00)00138-X

[74] Sripetchwandee J, Pipatpiboon N, Chattipakorn N, Chattipakorn S. Combined therapy of iron chelator and antioxidant completely restores brain dysfunction induced by iron toxicity. PLoS One. 2014;**9**:e85115. DOI: 10.1371/journal.pone.0085115

[75] Wongjaikam S, Kumfu S, Khamseekaew J, Sripetchwandee J, Srichairatanakool S, Fucharoen S, et al. Combined iron chelator and antioxidant exerted greater efficacy on cardioprotection than monotherapy in iron-overloaded rats. PLoS One. 2016;**11**:e0159414. DOI: 10.1371/journal.pone.0159414

[76] Imam MU, Zhang S, Ma J, Wang H, Wang F. Antioxidants Mediate Both Iron Homeostasis and Oxidative Stress. Nutrients. 2017;**9**(7):E671. DOI: 10.3390/nu9070671

[77] Vauzour D, Rodriguez-Mateos A, Corona G, Oruna-Concha MJ, Spencer JP. Polyphenols and human health: Prevention of disease and mechanisms of action. Nutrients. 2010;**2**:1106-1131. DOI: 10.3390/nu2111106

[78] Pandey KB, Rizvi SI. Plant polyphenols as dietary antioxidants in human health and disease. Oxidative Medicine and Cellular Longevity. 2009;**2**:270-278. DOI: 10.4161/oxim.2.5.9498

[79] Niu Q, Mu L, Li S, Xu S, Ma R, Guo S. Proanthocyanidin protects

human embryo hepatocytes from fluoride-induced oxidative stress by regulating iron metabolism. Biological Trace Element Research. 2016;**169**:174-179. DOI: 10.1007/s12011-015-0409-1

[80] Galati G, O'brien PJ. Potential toxicity of flavonoids and other dietary phenolics: Significance for their chemopreventive and anticancer properties. Free Radical Biology & Medicine. 2004;**37**:287-303. DOI: 10.1016/j.freeradbiomed.2004.04.034

[81] Zhong W, Qian K, Xiong J, Ma K, Wang A, Zou Y. Curcumin alleviates lipopolysaccharide induced sepsis and liver failure by suppression of oxidative stress-related inflammation via PI3K/AKT and NF-κB related signaling. Biomedicine & Pharmacotherapy. 2016;**83**:302-313. DOI: 10.1016/j.biopha.2016.06.036

[82] Zhao L, Wang Y, Liu J, Wang K, Guo X, Ji B, et al. Protective effects of genistein and puerarin against chronic alcohol-induced liver injury in mice via antioxidant, anti-inflammatory, and anti-apoptotic mechanisms. Journal of Agricultural and Food Chemistry. 2016;**64**:7291-7297. DOI: 10.1021/acs.jafc.6b02907

[83] Zhen AW, Nguyen NH, Gibert Y, Motola S, Buckett P, Wessling-Resnick M, et al. The small molecule, genistein, increases hepcidin expression in human hepatocytes. Hepatology. 2013;**58**:1315-1325. DOI: 10.1002/hep.26490

[84] MoayediEsfahani B, Reisi N, Mirmoghtadaei M. Evaluating the safety and efficacy of silymarin in β-thalassemia patients: A review. Hemoglobin. 2015;**39**:75-80. DOI: 10.3109/03630269.2014.1003224

[85] Kumar N, Pruthi V. Potential applications of ferulic acid from natural sources. Biotechnology Reports. 2014;**4**:86-93. DOI: 10.1016/j.btre.2014.09.002

[86] Bradamante S, Barenghi VA. Cardiovascular protective effects of resveratrol. Cardiovascular Drug Reviews. 2004;**22**:169-188. DOI: 10.1111/j.1527-3466.2004.tb00139.x.

[87] Tang PCT, Ng YF, Ho S, Gyda M, Chan SW. Resveratrol and cardiovascular health—Promising therapeutic or hopeless illusion? Pharmacological Research. 2014;**90**:88-115. DOI: 10.1016/j.phrs.2014.08.001

[88] McDowell LR, Wilkinson N, Madison R, Felix TL. Florida Ruminant Nutrition Symposium. Best Western Gateway Grand; Gainesville, FL, USA. Vitamins and minerals functioning as antioxidants with supplementation considerations2007. pp. 30-31

[89] García-Casal MN, Layrisse M, Solano L, Barón MA, Arguello F, Llovera D, et al. β-Carotene can improve non heme iron absorption from rice, wheat and corn by humans. The Journal of Nutrition. 1997;**128**:646-650

[90] Citelli M, Bittencourt LL, Da Silva SV, Pierucci AP, Pedrosa C. Vitamin a modulates the expression of genes involved in iron bioavailability. Biological Trace Element Research. 2012;**149**:64-70. DOI: 10.1007/s12011-012-9397-6

[91] Katz O, Reifen R, Lerner A. β-Carotene can reverse dysregulation of iron protein in an in vitro model of inflammation. Immunologic Research. 2015;**61**:70-78. DOI: 10.1007/s12026-014-8570-8

[92] Chiu PF, Ko SY, Chang CC. Vitamin C affects the expression of hepcidin and erythropoietin receptor in HepG2 cells. Journal of Renal Nutrition. 2012;**22**:373-376. DOI: 10.1053/j.jrn.2011.09.007

[93] Imam MU, Ismail M, Ooi DJ, Azmi NH, Sarega N, Chan KW, et al. Are bioactive-rich fractions functionally richer? Critical Reviews in Biotechnology. 2016;**36**:585-593

Chapter 7

Thromboembolism in Beta-Thalassemia Disease

Rungrote Natesirinilkul

Abstract

Thalassemia disease is a common inherited hemolytic anemia frequently found in several parts of the world, especially in the Mediterranean and some Asian countries. Besides the complications of secondary hemochromatosis from regular red blood cell (RBC) transfusion and increased gastrointestinal absorption of iron, thromboembolism (TE) is one of the common long-term complications of beta-thalassemia disease, particularly in patients with non-transfusion-dependent thalassemia (NTDT), which is commonly seen after the second decade of life. The risk factors of TE in beta-thalassemia disease including exposure of phosphatidylserine of abnormal RBCs, increase of platelet activation and aggregation, elevation of endothelial microparticles and increased endothelial activation, decreased nitric oxide (NO) secondary to hemolysis, rise of platelet count and nucleated RBCs after splenectomy, organ dysfunction caused by hemochromatosis, and thrombophilia such as natural anticoagulant deficiencies leading to hypercoagulable state. The understanding of the pathophysiology would result in effective prevention of this complication of beta-thalassemia disease.

Keywords: thromboembolism, beta-thalassemia, NTDT

1. Introduction

Beta-thalassemia disease is one of the most common congenital hemolytic anemia commonly found in the malarial belt areas including the Mediterranean, the Middle East, Transcaucasus, Africa, South and Southeast Asian countries, and China [1]. It is inherited by autosomal recessive manner [1, 2]. Beta-thalassemia disease is the result from the mutation of beta-globin genes causing decrease of beta-globin leading to imbalance of alpha-globin and beta-globin and subsequently causing ineffective erythropoiesis. According to the Thalassemia International Federation (TIF), patients with thalassemia disease can be categorized into two groups, transfusion-dependent thalassemia (TDT) and non-transfusion-dependent thalassemia (NTDT), based on their phenotypes and genotypes [1–3]. The major long-term complication of TDT is hemochromatosis-induced organ failures secondary to red blood cell (RBC) transfusion [1, 2], while the complications of NTDT are hemochromatosis secondary to increased iron absorption from gastrointestinal tract, pulmonary hypertension, leg ulcer, and thromboembolism (TE) [3–5].

The incidence of thromboembolism is between 0.8 and 2.7 per 1000 population [6] which has been increasing over the decades in both adult and pediatric population [6, 7] patients with thalassemia disease are at risk of hypercoagulable state and thromboembolism [8, 9]. The studies of thromboembolism in thalassemia disease have been increasingly published recently. Understanding the pathophysiology of thromboembolism in thalassemia diseases is the key for the management to prevent this complication.

2. Incidence

The incidence of thromboembolism in patients with thalassemia diseases is between 1.7 and 9.2% [4, 10, 11]; therefore, the incidence of thromboembolism in patients with thalassemia diseases is approximately 10 times higher than normal population [6]. The incidence is 4.4 times more prevalent in patients with NTDT than ones with TDT [10]. However, this complication could be seen in both patients alpha- and beta-thalassemia diseases [4].

3. Pathophysiology

The pathophysiology of thromboembolism in beta-thalassemia disease is the combinations of abnormalities in several parts of hemostatic system including [9, 12]:

1. Exposure of phosphatidylserine (PS) to external membrane of abnormal RBCs called "flip-flop phenomenon" which is caused by the decrease of normal asymmetrical dissemination of RBC membrane phospholipids [9]. In addition, free iron secondary to hemochromatosis induces lipid oxidation and elevates the level of membrane-bounded hemichromes and immunoglobulin causing alteration of the structures of spectrin and band 3 protein of RBC membrane and consequently resulting in aggregation and adhesion of abnormal RBCs to endothelial cells [9].

2. Increased number of circulating activated and aggregated platelets which are especially found in splenectomized patients [13, 14]. The activated and aggregated platelets of splenectomized patients with thalassemia usually have shorter platelet lifespan [14], higher response to several agonists, i.e., adenosine diphosphate (ADP), epinephrine, and collagen [15], and more elevated level of plasma beta-thromboglobulin [16] than the platelets of normal population. All findings reflect hyperaggregation of platelets which result in increased thrombin generation [15].

3. Increased endothelial activation caused by the activation of monocytes and granulocytes leads to endothelial injury and increased level of endothelial adhesion proteins and tissue factor contributing to hypercoaguable state. Moreover, the elevation of endothelial cell, platelet and white blood cell (WBC) and RBC microparticles, which are the shedded fragments containing high PS with the size of 0.1–2 μm from activated and apoptotic cells, leads to increased activation of hemostatic system [17–19].

4. Decreased nitric oxide (NO), secondary to hemolysis caused by the decreased level of arginine leads to pulmonary vasoconstriction and subsequently results in chronic pulmonary thromboembolism [12, 20].

5. Rise of platelet count and nucleated RBCs (NRBCs) after splenectomy which was firstly reported in 1966 [21]. This phenomenon is a strong associated factor of thromboembolism in patients with thalassemia disease particularly

when the platelet count is higher than 600,000/mm^3 and the NRBCs count is more than 300/mm^3 after splenectomy [22].

6. Organ dysfunction resulting from hemochromatosis particularly cardiac hemochromatosis causes cardiomyopathy and cardiac arrhythmia [12] which is found in beta-thalassemic patients who TDT for 42% [23].

7. Thrombophilia, i.e., natural anticoagulant deficiencies, leads to hypercoagulable state. Deficiencies of protein C and protein S, the natural anticoagulant proteins, have been reported as a risk factor of thromboembolism in patients with beta-thalassemia disease [12, 24, 25]. In addition, increased incidence of antiphospholipid antibodies, i.e., lupus anticoagulant, anticardiolipin, and anti-beta 2-glycoprotein 1, is commonly found in patients with beta-thalassemia disease. Those antibodies are considered as strong thrombophilic risk factors causing thromboembolism [12, 26].

4. Presentations of thromboembolism in beta-thalassemia

Thromboembolism in patients with beta-thalassemia diseases could be found in both arterial and venous sites. However, venous thromboembolism is more commonly found in patients with thalassemia intermedia or NTDT, while arterial thromboembolism is more frequently seen in patients with thalassemia major or TDT [10].

4.1 Venous thromboembolism

Although patients with beta-thalassemia disease are at risk of venous thromboembolism, deep vein thrombosis and pulmonary thromboembolism, the two common types of venous thromboembolism in normal population, are not generally observed. Pulmonary thromboembolism was found in lung biopsy to 41% of patients with beta-thalassemia/hemoglobin E. However, higher incidence was found in the older and splenectomized patients [27]. Simplified, revised Geneva score, based on several clinical variables, i.e., hemoptysis, old age of more than 65 years, history of venous thromboembolism, tachycardia, unilateral lower limb pain with or without deep palpation and edema, active malignancy, and surgery or fracture of lower limb within 1 month prior to the suspected symptoms and signs, has been published to use for diagnosing pulmonary thromboembolism. The more scores patients get, the higher chance of pulmonary embolism patients have [28]. Computed tomography pulmonary angiography, magnetic resonance pulmonary angiography, and ventilation/perfusion scan could be used to diagnose pulmonary thromboembolism even though conventional pulmonary angiography is the gold standard [29].

Portal vein thrombosis, which is considered as venous thrombosis of an unusual site, is more commonly reported in patients with beta-thalassemia disease [30–34] with the odds ratio of 3.5 [31]. Patients with acute portal vein thrombosis usually present with symptoms and signs of portal hypertension of bowel ischemia, i.e., abdominal pain and distension, fever, nausea/vomiting, rectal hemorrhage, and splenomegaly. If patients were not diagnosed, they might turn to sepsis-like symptoms, e.g., shock, signs of peritonitis, and even death [35]. Unlike acute portal vein thrombosis, patients with chronic portal vein thrombosis are usually asymptomatic until the presence of first symptoms and signs, i.e., upper gastrointestinal hemorrhage, splenomegaly, and ascites [35]. Doppler ultrasound, computed tomography, and magnetic resonance imaging could be used for diagnosis of portal vein thrombosis [35]. Apart from splenectomy, higher splenic weight and thalassemia intermedia are major risk factors of portal vein thrombosis in patients with beta-thalassemia disease [30, 33]. Laparoscopic splenectomy was reported about the higher incidence of portal vein thrombosis even though this technique provided the better other surgical outcomes than the conventional technique [30].

4.2 Arterial ischemic stroke

Beta-thalassemia disease has been reported as a risk factor of arterial ischemic stroke since 1972 [36]. Compared to venous thromboembolism, arterial ischemic stroke is more common in patients with beta-thalassemia major [11]. Moyamoya syndrome, a cerebral vasculopathy caused by spontaneous occlusion of the arteries at the circle of Willis [37], was also reported in pediatric patients with beta-thalassemia disease and caused arterial ischemic stroke [38, 39]. Symptom and signs of acute ischemic stroke are based on the involved cerebral areas ranging from nonspecific symptoms, i.e., headache, nausea and vomiting, seizure, and impaired consciousness to specific neurological deficits, i.e., abnormal speech and spatial perception, hemiparesis, hemianesthesia, blurred vision, and poor coordination or walking, and cranial nerve palsies [40]. Though computed tomography of the head with or without angiography is the standard for diagnosing arterial ischemic stroke, magnetic resonance imaging of head with or without angiography could provide more details of the affected parts of the brain with higher sensitivity [40].

Moreover, the focal foci in the cerebral white matter on the magnetic resonance imaging of the brain called "silent cerebral infarction" could be found at 24–61% of patients with beta-thalassemia disease [41, 42]. However, a recent study in adult patients with beta-thalassemia disease who were asymptomatic showed that the abnormal findings on the magnetic resonance imaging of the brain were not different from the adult controls [43].

4.3 Diagnosis

Making a diagnosis of thromboembolism in patients with beta-thalassemia does not differ from diagnosing this condition in normal population which is usually based on the imaging of the suspected area of thromboembolism, e.g., computed tomography with angiography of the brain in a patient who is suspicious for having an arterial ischemic stroke. Several studies have demonstrated derangement of proteins hemostatic system in patients with beta-thalassemia diseases including increased platelet aggregation and coagulation proteins (factor VIII and von Willebrand factor) and decreased natural anticoagulants (protein C, protein S, and antithrombin) [24, 25] which encourage hypercoagulable state [44]. Besides diagnosing a symptomatic patient, the novel investigations, i.e., thrombin generation assay and rotatory thromboelastometry (ROTEM®), are able to demonstrate patients with hypercoagulable state in patients with beta-thalassemia disease who are at risk of developing thromboembolism [45, 46]. In addition, yearly monitoring of thrombin generation markers, e.g., D-dimer and thrombin-antithrombin (TAT) complex, is recommended by TIF in patients with thalassemia who are splenectomized [47].

5. Treatment

1. Regular RBC transfusion is recommended to treat patients with beta-thalassemia disease, particularly NTDT, who are at risk of thromboembolism or have developed thromboembolic events by keeping hemoglobin level higher

than 9 g/dL [3] to correct hypercoagulable state as transfusion naïve patients are prone to have thromboembolism [12, 22, 48].

2. Hematopoietic stem cell transplantation (HSCT) has been reported as the management that could normalize the abnormal hemostatic derangement in patients with beta-thalassemia disease by increasing natural anticoagulant proteins and decreasing microparticles and RBC-expressing PS and activating platelets in the circulation [49, 50].

3. Antithrombotic agents in patients with beta-thalassemia disease who have thromboembolism are recommended as per the standard local or international guidelines to treat patients with thromboembolism [3, 12].

    a. Anti-platelets: acetyl salicylic acid (ASA)

ASA 2–5 mg/kg/day is the mainstream management for the prevention and treatment of thromboembolism in patients in beta-thalassemia especially in splenectomized patients who have platelet count higher than 500,000/mm^3 [3]. However, ASA resistance has been reported in patients with thalassemia who were splenectomized, and increase dose of ASA could overcome this resistance [51].

    b. Anticoagulants consist of conventional anticoagulants, i.e., unfractionated heparin, low-molecular-weight heparin, vitamin K antagonist (VKA), and direct oral anticoagulants (DOAC) including direct oral anti-activated factor X (Xa), e.g., rivaroxaban, and direct oral antithrombin (IIa), i.e. dabigratan. Those medications are used to treat thromboembolism in patients with beta-thalassemia disease. Unlike sickle cell disease, the evidences of using DOAC in patients with thalassemia disease who develop thromboembolism are limited [52]. However, the recent study showed that using rivaroxaban in patients with hemoglobinopathies including thalassemia was effective and did not increase risk of bleeding or thrombosis [53].

4. Hydroxyurea, a hemoglobin F stimulating agent, was reported about the favorable effects not only increased hemoglobin F, hemoglobin level and improved the clinical symptoms of beta-thalassemia disease but also decreased hypercoagulable state due to the diminished exposure of PS on RBC membrane [54, 55]. Moreover, Iqbal et al. recently reported the change of metabolites, i.e., glycerol, triethanolamine, linoleic acid, palmitic acid, and stearic acid to the healthy pattern of metabolic pathway in pediatric patients with beta-thalassemia disease after treating with hydroxyurea [56].

Since patients with beta-thalassemia disease are at risk of thromboembolism as the same as other medical inpatients, the current approach is to stratify patients with the optimal risk assessment model (RAM) by using the available approaches, e.g., Padua Prediction Score and the Caprini Risk Assessment Model, to guide thromboprophylaxis [57]. However, the systematic review showed that there was not any specific risk assessment model which was superior to the others [58]. Moreover, thalassemia-specific risk assessment model for thromboprophylaxis may need to be developed due to distinctive pathophysiology of thromboembolism in patients with beta-thalassemia disease.

In conclusion, the hypercoagulable state in beta-thalassemia disease is the result of several risk factors, a combination of which is often the drive behind a clinical thromboembolism. Splenectomy and transfusion naivety are increasingly highlighted as important risk factors for thromboembolism, especially in patients with NTDT. An individualized approach is recommended to establish an optimal strategy for preventing the occurrence of this complication in patients with beta-thalassemia disease.

Author details

Rungrote Natesirinilkul
Division of Hematology and Oncology, Department of Pediatrics, Faculty of Medicine, Chiang Mai University, Thailand

*Address all correspondence to: rungrote.n@cmu.ac.th

References

[1] Viprakasit V, Origa R. Genetic basis, pathophysiology and diagnosis. In: Cappellini MD, Cohen A, Porter J, Taher A, Viprakasit V, editors. Guidelines for the Management of Transfusion Dependent Thalassaemia (TDT). 3rd ed. Nicosia: Thalassaemia International Federation; 2014. pp. 14-27

[2] Viprakasit V, Ekwattanakit S. Clinical classification, screening and diagnosis for thalassemia. Hematology/Oncology Clinics of North America. 2018;**32**:193-211

[3] Taher A, Musallam K, Cappellini MD. Guidelines for the Management of Non Transfusion Dependent Thalassaemia (NTDT). 2nd ed. Nicosia: Thalassaemia International Federation; 2017

[4] Winichakoon P, Tantiworawit A, Rattanathammethee T, Hantrakool S, Chai-Adisaksopha C, Rattarittamrong E, et al. Prevalence and risk factors for complications in patients with nontransfusion dependent alpha- and beta-thalassemia. Anemia. 2015;**2015**:793025. DOI: 10.1155/2015/793025

[5] Teawtrakul N, Jetsrisuparb A, Pongudom S, Sirijerachai C, Chansung K, Wanitpongpun C, et al. Epidemiologic study of major complications in adolescent and adult patients with thalassemia in Northeastern Thailand: The E-SAAN study phase I. Hematology. 2018;**23**:55-60

[6] ISTH Steering Committee for World Thrombosis Day. Thrombosis: A major contributor to the global disease burden. Journal of Thrombosis and Haemostasis. 2014;**12**:1580-1590

[7] Raffini L, Huang YS, Witmer C, Feudtner C. Dramatic increase in venous thromboembolism in children's hospitals in the United States from 2001 to 2007. Pediatrics. 2009;**124**:1001-1008

[8] Taher AT, Musallam KM, Inati A. The hypercoagulable state in thalassemia intermedia. Hemoglobin. 2009;**33**:160-169

[9] Eldor A, Rachmilewitz EA. The hypercoagulable state in thalassemia. Blood. 2002;**99**:36-43

[10] Taher A, Isma'eel H, Mehio G, Bignamini D, Kattamis A, Rachmilewitz EA, et al. Prevalence of thromboembolic events among 8,860 patients with thalassaemia major and intermedia in the Mediterranean area and Iran. Thrombosis and Haemostasis. 2006;**96**:488-491

[11] Borgna pignatti C, Carnelli V, Caruso V, Dore F, De Mattia D, Di Palma A, et al. Thromboembolic events in beta thalassemia major: An Italian multicenter study. Acta Haematologica. 1998;**99**:76-79

[12] Sirachainan N. Thalassemia and the hypercoagulable state. Thrombosis Research. 2013;**132**:637-641

[13] Winichagoon P, Fucharoen S, Wasi P. Increased circulating platelet aggregates in thalassaemia. The Southeast Asian Journal of Tropical Medicine and Public Health. 1981;**12**:556-560

[14] Eldor A, Krausz Y, Atlan H, Snyder D, Goldfarb A, Hy-Am E, et al. Platelet survival in patients with beta-thalassemia. American Journal of Hematology. 1989;**32**:94-99

[15] Visudhiphan S, Ketsa-Ard K, Tumliang S, Piankijagum A. Significance of blood coagulation and platelet profiles in relation to pulmonary thrombosis in beta-thalassemia/Hb E. Southeast Asian Journal of

Tropical Medicine and Public Health. 1994;**25**:449-456

[16] Atichartakarn V, Angchaisuksiri P, Aryurachai K, Chuncharunee S, Thakkinstian A. In vivo platelet activation and hyperaggregation in hemoglobin E/beta-thalassemia: A consequence of splenectomy. International Journal of Hematology. 2003;77:299-303

[17] Agouti I, Cointe S, Robert S, Judicone C, Loundou A, Driss F, et al. Plateletandnoterythrocytemicroparticles are procoagulant in transfused thalassaemia major patients. British Journal of Haematology. 2015;**171**:615-624

[18] Youssry I, Soliman N, Ghamrawy M, Samy RM, Nasr A, Abdel Mohsen M, et al. Circulating microparticles and the risk of thromboembolic events in Egyptian beta thalassemia patients. Annals of Hematology. 2017;**96**:597-603

[19] Klaihmon P, Phongpao K, Kheansaard W, Noulsri E, Khuhapinant A, Fucharoen S, et al. Microparticles from splenectomized β-thalassemia/HbE patients play roles on procoagulant activities with thrombotic potential. Annals of Hematology. 2017;**96**:189-198

[20] Tantawy AA, Adly AA, Ismail EA, Aly SH. Endothelial nitric oxide synthase gene intron 4 variable number tandem repeat polymorphism in β-thalassemia major: Relation to cardiovascular complications. Blood Coagulation & Fibrinolysis. 2015;**26**:419-425

[21] Hirsh J, Dacie JV. Persistent post-splenectomy thrombocytosis and thrombo-embolism: A consequence of continuing anaemia. British Journal of Haematology. 1966;**12**:44-53

[22] Taher AT, Musallam KM, Karimi M, El-Beshlawy A, Belhoul K, Daar S, et al. Splenectomy and thrombosis: The case of thalassemia intermedia. Journal of Thrombosis and Haemostasis. 2010;**8**:2152-2158

[23] Koohi F, Kazemi T, Miri-Moghaddam E. Cardiac complications and iron overload in beta thalassemia major patients—A systematic review and meta-analysis. Annals of Hematology. 2019;**98**:1323-1331

[24] Huang Y, Long Y, Deng D, Liu Z, Liang H, Sun N, et al. Alterations of anticoagulant proteins and soluble endothelial protein C receptor in thalassemia patients of Chinese origin. Thrombosis Research. 2018;**172**:61-66

[25] Angchaisuksiri P, Atichartakarn V, Aryurachai K, Archararit N, Chuncharunee S, Tiraganjana A, et al. Hemostatic and thrombotic markers in patients with hemoglobin E/beta-thalassemia disease. American Journal of Hematology. 2007;**82**:1001-1004

[26] Sharma S, Raina V, Chandra J, Narayan S, Sharma S. Lupus anticoagulant and anticardiolipin antibodies in polytransfused beta thalassemia major. Hematology. 2006;**11**:287-290

[27] Sonakul D, Fucharoen S. Pulmonary thromboembolism in thalassemic patients. The Southeast Asian Journal of Tropical Medicine and Public Health. 1992;**23**:25-28

[28] Kline JA, Ellison AM, Kanis J, Pike JW, Hall CL. Evaluation of the pulmonary embolism rule out criteria (PERC rule) in children evaluated for suspected pulmonary embolism. Thrombosis Research. 2018;**168**:1-4

[29] Yui V, Natesirinilkul R, Brandao LR. Disordered hemostasis and renal disorders. In: Geary DF, Schaefer F, editors. Pediatric Kidney Disease. 2nd ed. Berlin: Springer; 2016. pp. 799-834

[30] Wang M, Zhang M, Li J, Zhou J, Wu Z, Peng B. Risk factors of portal vein thrombosis in patients with beta thalassemia major after splenectomy: Laparoscopic versus open procedure. Hepato-Gastroenterology. 2014;**61**:48-54

[31] Sabbagh A, Keikhaei B, Joorabian M, Behzad MM, Momeni M. Retrospective study of the incidence of portal vein thrombosis after splenectomy in hematological disorders: Risk factors and clinical presentation. Blood Cells, Molecules & Diseases. 2019;**74**:1-4

[32] Alexakis N, Dardamanis D, Albanopoulos K, Ptohis N, Skalistira M, Karagiorga M, et al. Incidence, risk factors, and outcome of portal vein thrombosis after laparoscopic-assisted splenectomy in β-thalassemia patients: A prospective exploratory study. Journal of Laparoendoscopic & Advanced Surgical Techniques. Part A. 2013;**23**:123-128

[33] Elalfy MS, Andrawes NG, Sadek AM, Hussein O, Abdou A. D-dimer and portal vein status in splenectomized Egyptian β-thalassemia major patients: A prospective single-thalassemia center experience. Pediatric Hematology and Oncology. 2012;**29**:247-253

[34] Hassan MN, Tahereb GM, Ahmad T, Asghar DA, Reza ED, Ali B, et al. Correlation of splenectomy with portal vein thrombosis in beta-thalassemia major. The Journal of the Pakistan Medical Association. 2011;**61**:760-762

[35] Ponziani FR, Zocco MA, Campanale C, Rinninella E, Tortora A, Di Maurizio L, et al. Portal vein thrombosis: Insight into physiopathology, diagnosis, and treatment. World Journal of Gastroenterology. 2010;**16**:143-155

[36] Logothetis J, Constantoulakis M, Economidou J, Stefanis C, Hakas P, Augoustaki O, et al. Thalassemia major (homozygous beta-thalassemia). A survey of 138 cases with emphasis on neurologic and muscular aspects. Neurology. 1972;**22**:294-304

[37] Scott RM, Smith ER. Moyamoya disease and moyamoya syndrome. The New England Journal of Medicine. 2009;**360**:1226-1237

[38] Oberoi S, Bansal D, Singh P, Marwaha RK. Stroke in a young boy with β-thalassemia intermedia secondary to moyamoya syndrome. Journal of Pediatric Hematology/Oncology. 2010;**32**:568-570

[39] Marden FA, Putman CM, Grant JM, Greenberg J. Moyamoya disease associated with hemoglobin Fairfax and beta-thalassemia. Pediatric Neurology. 2008;**38**:130-132

[40] Musuka TD, Wilton SB, Traboulsi M, Hill MD. Diagnosis and management of acute ischemic stroke: Speed is critical. CMAJ. 2015;**187**:887-893

[41] Pazgal I, Inbar E, Cohen M, Shpilberg O, Stark P. High incidence of silent cerebral infarcts in adult patients with beta thalassemia major. Thrombosis Research. 2016;**144**:119-122

[42] Metarugcheep P, Chanyawattiwongs S, Srisubat K, Pootrakul P. Clinical silent cerebral infarct (SCI) in patients with thalassemia diseases assessed by magnetic resonance imaging (MRI). Journal of the Medical Association of Thailand. 2008;**91**:889-894

[43] Tartaglione I, Russo C, Elefante A, Caiazza M, Casale M, Di Concilio R, et al. No evidence of increased cerebrovascular involvement in adult neurologically-asymptomatic β-thalassaemia. A multicentre multimodal magnetic resonance study. British Journal of Haematology. 2019;**185**:733-742

[44] Tripatara A, Jetsrisuparb A, Teeratakulpisarn J, Kuaha K. Hemostatic alterations in splenectomized and non-splenectomized patients with beta-thalassemia/hemoglobin E disease. Thrombosis Research. 2007;**120**:805-810

[45] Tripodi A, Cappellini MD, Chantarangkul V, Padovan L, Fasulo MR, Marcon A, et al. Hypercoagulability in splenectomized thalassemic patients detected by whole-blood thromboelastometry, but not by thrombin generation in platelet-poor plasma. Haematologica. 2009;**94**:1520-1527

[46] Natesirinilkul R, Charoenkwan P, Nawarawong W, Boonsri S, Tantivate P, Wongjaikum S, et al. Hypercoagulable state as demonstrated by thromboelastometry in hemoglobin E/ beta-thalassemia patients: Association with clinical severity and splenectomy status. Thrombosis Research. 2016;**140**:125-131

[47] Taher A, Tyan PI. The spleen. In: Cappellini MD, Cohen A, Porter J, Taher A, Viprakasit V, editors. Guidelines for the Management of Transfusion Dependent Thalassaemia (TDT). 3rd ed. Nicosia: Thalassaemia International Federation; 2014. pp. 126-133

[48] Atichartakarn V, Chuncharunee S, Chandanamattha P, Likittanasombat K, Aryurachai K. Correction of hypercoagulability and amelioration of pulmonary arterial hypertension by chronic blood transfusion in an asplenic hemoglobin E/beta-thalassemia patient. Blood. 2004;**103**:2844-2846

[49] Sirachainan N, Thongsad J, Pakakasama S, Hongeng S, Chuansumrit A, Kadegasem P, et al. Normalized coagulation markers and anticoagulation proteins in children with severe β-thalassemia disease after stem cell transplantation. Thrombosis Research. 2012;**129**:765-770

[50] Klaihmon P, Vimonpatranon S, Noulsri E, Lertthammakiat S, Anurathapan U, Sirachainan N, et al. Normalized levels of red blood cells expressing phosphatidylserine, their microparticles, and activated platelets in young patients with β-thalassemia following bone marrow transplantation. Annals of Hematology. 2017;**96**:1741-1747

[51] Sirachainan N, Wijarn P, Chuansumrit A, Kadegasem P, Wongwerawattanakoon P, Soisamrong A. Aspirin resistance in children and young adults with splenectomized thalassemia diseases. Thrombosis Research. 2015;**135**:916-922

[52] Shet AS, Wun T. How I diagnose and treat venous thromboembolism in sickle cell disease. Blood. 2018;**132**:1761-1769

[53] Apostolou C, Klonizakis P, Mainou M, Kapsali E, Kafantari K, Kotsiafti A, et al. Rivaroxaban use in patients with hemoglobinopathies. Hemoglobin. 2017;**41**:223-224

[54] Musallam KM, Taher AT, Cappellini MD, Sankaran VG. Clinical experience with fetal hemoglobin induction therapy in patients with β-thalassemia. Blood. 2013;**121**:2199-2212

[55] Musallam KM, Taher AT. Thrombosis in thalassemia: Why are we so concerned? Hemoglobin. 2011;**35**:503-510

[56] Iqbal A, Ansari SH, Parveen S, Khan IA, Siddiqui AJ, Musharraf SG. Hydroxyurea treated β-thalassemia children demonstrate a shift in metabolism towards healthy pattern. Scientific Reports. 2018;**8**:15152

[57] Zhou H, Hu Y, Xiaoqian Li X, Wang L, Wang M, Xiao J, et al. Assessment of the risk of venous thromboembolism in medical inpatients using the Padua prediction score and

Caprini risk assessment model. Journal of Atherosclerosis and Thrombosis. 2018;**25**:1091-1104

[58] Stuck AK, Spirk D, Schaudt J, Kucher N. Risk assessment models for venous thromboembolism in acutely ill medical patients. A systematic review. Thrombosis and Haemostasis. 2017;**117**:801-808

Section 4

Diagnosis of Beta Thalassemia

Chapter 8

Laboratory Diagnosis of β-Thalassemia and HbE

Thanusak Tatu

Abstract

β-Thalassemia and HbE, each, is a syndrome resulted from quantitative and qualitative defects of β-globin chain, respectively. In addition to history retrieve and physical examination, diagnosis of these disorders requires laboratory information. Laboratory tests that are conventionally performed to diagnose the β-thalassemia and HbE are classified into two groups, based on the purposes, including the screening tests and confirmatory tests. The screening tests are aimed to screen for carriers of the β-thalassemia and HbE, while confirmatory tests are the tests performed to definitely diagnose these disorders. This chapter will explain all of these tests, the information of which will be useful for those who are working and interested in the β-thalassemia and HbE.

Keywords: β-thalassemia, HbE, screening tests, confirmatory tests, thalassemia carrier, HbE carrier, β-thalassemia disease

1. Introduction

1.1 Thalassemia and hemoglobinopathies

Thalassemia is a type of anemia caused by reduction or absence of globin chain synthesis, which results in imbalanced-globin chain synthesis; the major pathogenesis of the disease. The unaffected globin chains continuing to be synthesized at the normal synthetic rate tend to form homotetramers and aggregation that can harm the red blood cells both at young and mature stages. The α-globin chain aggregation formed in β-thalassemia causes ineffective erythropoiesis due to oxidative stress. The γ- and β-globin chain homotetramer (γ_4, β_4) formed in α-thalassemia harm mature erythrocytes. The γ_4 or Hb Bart's has very high oxygen affinity and inhibits oxygen release from erythrocytes which, in turn, results in tissue anoxia. The β4 or HbH is an unstable hemoglobin and precipitates easily under the stress condition in the body. Once precipitates, the erythrocytes are removed by the RE system resulting in anemia.

Severe thalassemia cases suffer from chronic and marked anemia with life relying solely on blood transfusion. Anemia causes expansion of bone marrow, leading to osteoporosis and changes of bone structure. Blood transfusion and hemolysis cause iron overloading state in the body which causes several complications such as heart disease, growth retardation, diabetes mellitus, and infection.

Thalassemia is considered the most common autosomal single-gene disorder worldwide. It can be found in more than 150 countries with an estimated carrier frequency of about 7%. The Mediterranean region, certain parts of North and West Africa, Middle East, Indian subcontinent, Southern Far East, and South East Asia have the highest prevalence of the disease [1].

In contrast to the thalassemia, hemoglobinopathy is an inherited disorder of hemoglobin productions characterized by production of abnormal hemoglobin or hemoglobin structural variants occurring from genetic alterations including point mutations, deletions or insertion of the normal globin genes. The well-known abnormal hemoglobins in the world are HbS, which is common in western countries as well as in the Middle East and HbE, which is common in Southeast Asia [2].

1.2 Types of thalassemia and hemoglobinopathies

Two major types of thalassemia are found across the world consisting of the α- and β-thalassemia. The α-thalassemia is further sub-divided into two types: α-thalassemia 1 or α^{O}-thalassemia and α-thalassemia 2 or α^{+}-thalassemia. Gene deletion is the leading cause of α-thalassemia. In α-thalassemia 1, two α-globin gene in-cis on chromosome 16 are deleted, while only one α-globin gene is absent in the α-thalassemia 2 [3]. In addition, there are two types of β-thalassemia; β^{O}-thalassemia and β^{+}-thalassemia. In contrast to α-thalassemia, mutations on the β-globin gene are found in the majority of the β-thalassemia patients [4].

Two broad types of hemoglobinopathies or structural variants are also found; α- and β-hemoglobinopathies. To date, approximately 1358 structural variants are described (http://globin.bx.psu.edu), around 90% of which are involved in the β, γ, and δ-globin chains and around 60% involves the α-globin chain. The most important β-globin hemoglobinopathies are HbS ($\alpha_2\beta_2^{6Glu-Val}$) and HbE ($\alpha^2\beta_2^{26Glu-Lys}$). Hb E is found around the world and accounts for approximately 13–17% on the population of Thailand, especially in the Thai-Laos-Cambodian boundary or "Hb E triangle" where more than 32–60% of the people carry HbE gene [5].

1.2.1 β-Thalassemia

The β-thalassemia is a diverse group of disorders of hemoglobin synthesis which is characterized by reduced or absent β-globin chain synthesis. There are two main types of β-thalassemia: β^{O}-thalassemia in which no β-globin chain is produced and β^{+}-thalassemia in which some β-globin is produced but less than normal.

β^{0}-Thalassemia is severe β-thalassemia with no production of β-globin chain. It is mainly caused by point mutations in coding region (exon) or exon-intron junction of β-globin gene which lead to premature stop codon or generation of abnormal β-globin mRNA. The end results of these abnormalities are absence of the β-globin chain production [6]. In Thailand, at least three common mutations in the β-globin gene are of this category. They comprise A-T substitution at codon 17 (CD17: A-T) which creates premature stop codon, the TTCT-deletion at codons 41/42 (CD41/42: –TTCT) which causes reading frameshift and premature stop codon at codon 59 instead of codon 147, the G-T substitution at IVSI-nt1 which leads to abnormal splicing of immature β-mRNA and results in no production of normal β-mRNA. In general, thus, genotype of heterozygote is written as β^{0}/β^{A} and that for homozygote as β^{0}/β^{0} [2, 7–9].

β^{+}-Thalassemia is a milder form of β-thalassemia in which some β-globin chains are still produced. The majority of cases possess point mutations outside exons, especially in the promoter region. The mutations of β-globin gene leading to the β^{+}-thalassemia include mutations at ATA box (nt-28, nt-29 or nt-30 from cap site), CACCC element (nt-86 to nt-90 from cap site), and mutations in introns or exons of gene to produce new splice site to race in RNA splicing process, as mutation in IVS2-nt654 (C-T) and mutation of IVS1-nt5 (G-C) [2, 6]. The genotypes were β^{+}/β^{A} and β^{+}/β^{+} for heterozygote and homozygote consecutively.

1.2.2 β-Hemoglobinopathies

β-Hemoglobinopathies are characterized by the production of abnormal β-globin chains due to changes or mutations (missense mutations) on the β-globin gene. Two abnormal β-globin chains then assemble with two normal α-globin chains to form abnormal hemoglobin or β-structural variants. These abnormal hemoglobins generally have different electrophysical properties from their normal counterparts; that is, due to the molecular conformational alteration. In theory, synthetic rate of the abnormal β-globin chain should be normal. However, some are produced in reduced rate, thus producing a phenotype resembling the β^{+}-thalassemia. To date, there are more than 737 β-globin structural variants reports across the world (http://globin.cse.psu.edu/).

1.3 Hemoglobin E

HbE is abnormal hemoglobin resulted from the G-A substitution at codon 26 of β-globin gene. This missense mutation partially activates a cryptic splice site toward the 3′ end of exon 1, resulting in a proportion of abnormally splice mRNA. Thus, less β^{E} globin is synthesized, leading to a mild thalassemia phenotype. HbE is becoming the common β-globin structure variant across the world as a result of migration and inter racial marriage [2, 10]. It has been realized to be the hallmark of Southeast Asian region. In Thailand, HbE is very common accounting for approximately 8–70% of population [11].

1.4 Inheritance of genes for β-thalassemia and HbE

Gene for β-thalassemia and HbE is transmitted within the family from parents to descendants in an autosomal recessive fashion. Thus, those who are heterozygous for abnormal β-gene are clinically asymptomatic and called β-thalassemia carrier or β-thalassemia trait. Those who are heterozygote for HbE gene (β^{E}) are also clinically asymptomatic and called HbE carrier or HbE trait. However, homozygote or compound heterozygote of the β-thalassemia gene and/or HbE gene are clinically affected and suffer from chronic anemia with some life-threatening complication. Therefore, accurate diagnosis of carriers of the β-thalassemia and HbE as well as the disease is important.

1.5 Problem of β-thalassemia and HbE

The carriers of β-thalassemia and HbE do not have clinical burden as they are clinically normal and have normal quality of life. However, if the β-thalassemia carriers get married with the HbE carriers, they will have 25% chance of producing the HbE/β-thalassemia babies. The HbE/β-thalassemia or sometimes called the β-thalassemia/HbE disease is a thalassemia syndrome that presently is known to be clinically heterogeneous [10–12]. Some patients are very mild, while some are very severe. The severe cases always required regular blood transfusion which always ends up with iron overloading condition. Without proper management of this iron overloading, several fatal complications occur, leading to low quality of life and, finally, pre-death at young age.

1.6 Diagnosis of β-thalassemia and HbE

The diagnosis of β-thalassemia and HbE involves both clinical and laboratory investigations. Clinical data can only identify the affected patients, but cannot definitely identify types of thalassemia the patients are suffering. Laboratory data thus help define specific types of thalassemia disease of those affected individuals. For the carriers, as they are clinically normal, clinical data are of no use. Only laboratory data can define β-thalassemia and HbE carriers.

Conventionally, the laboratory tests for diagnosis of β-thalassemia and HbE include screening tests and confirmatory tests. Initial screening tests are defined as techniques that are simple and relatively low cost, which can indicate the possibility of having thalassemia. These tests should involve the least sample pretreatment and rapid sample preparation and may not need special instrumentation. This would lead to low cost and high sample throughput analysis. The screening tests, however, cannot provide the information on the exact type of thalassemia of the positive persons. Positive samples need further confirmatory test while negative samples can be eliminated from further complicated and expensive testing.

The screening tests for β-thalassemia carriers comprise one-tube osmotic fragility test (OFT) and automated red blood cell indices (mean corpuscular volume; MCV, mean corpuscular hemoglobin; MCH, and red cell distribution width; RDW). Screening tests for HbE carriers are composed of all tests performed to screen for the β-thalassemia carrier plus the specifically established for HbE screen such as dichlorophenolindophenol precipitation (DCIP) test or HbE tube test or HbE test [13–16]. These screening tests, however, cannot provide the information on the exact type of thalassemia of the positive persons.

The purpose and methodologies of confirmatory tests for β-thalassemia and HbE are identical. The confirmatory tests must be highly specific in order to obtain the correct diagnosis of carriers of β-thalassemia and HbE as well as the disease state of HbE/β-thalassemia and homozygote or compound heterozygote of the β-thalassemia gene. The confirmatory tests include;

- Hemoglobin studies: Tests for hemoglobin studies include cellulose acetate electrophoresis, microcolumn chromatography, alkaline denaturation test, cation-exchange high performance liquid chromatography (HPLC) [17–19], cation-exchange low pressure liquid chromatography (LPLC) [20–22], capillary zone electrophoresis (CZE) [23–27], sandwich enzyme linked immunosorbent assay (ELISA) for Hb F [28], Hb Bart's [29] and Hb A_2 [30], flow cytometric analysis of F cells [31], and immunochromatographic strip (IC strip) test for Hb Bart's [32].

- DNA analysis: Tests for analysis of β-globin gene mutations include multiplex allele-specific polymerase chain reaction (MAS-PCR) [29], amplification refractory mutation system (ARMS)-PCR [33], mutagenically separated (MS)-PCR [34–36], and high resolution melting curve (HRM) analysis [37–39].

2. Screening laboratory tests for β-thalassemia and HbE carriers

Two laboratory tests are usually performed for screening of the β-thalassemia carriers: automated red cell indices (mean corpuscular volume; MCV, mean corpuscular hemoglobin; MCH, and red cell distribution width; RDW) and one-tube osmotic fragility test (OFT). The screening tests for HbE carrier comprise those performed for the β-thalassemia screen plus the tests used for HbE screen. These tests include dichlorophenolindophenol precipitation (DCIP) test [40], HbE-tube test [15], and hemoglobin E test [16]. The results of these screening tests indicate chance that the blood samples are carriers of either β-thalassemia or HbE.

2.1 Red blood cell indices

Red blood cells or erythrocyte indices used for screening for β-thalassemia carriers and HbE carriers conventionally included mean corpuscular volume (MCV) and mean corpuscular hemoglobin (MCH). These red cell indices must be obtained by automated blood cell analyzers. Normal ranges of MCV and MCH are 85.5 ± 6.8 fL and 27.1 ± 3.1 pg, respectively. Cut-off points of MCV and MCH are 80 fL and 27 pg, respectively.

MCV and MCH in β-thalassemia carriers are 68.7 ± 5.4 fL and 20.6 ± 2.1 pg. In HbE carriers, MCV and MCH values are 76.3 ± 4.6 fL and 24.2 ± 1.5 pg [41]. We found that the MCV and MCH in normal individuals, β-thalassemia carriers, and HbE carriers were significantly different [41]. With the cut-off points of 80 fL, MCV has been shown to be effective in screening for the β-thalassemia carriers with sensitivity and specificity of 92.9 and 83.9%, respectively [42, 43]. At 26.5 pg cut-off point of MCH, Pranpanus and co-workers found 92.5% sensitivity and 83.2% specificity of MCH in screening for the β-thalassemia carriers. At the cut-off point of 80 fL for MCV and 27 pg for MCH, Karimi and co-workers found 98.5% sensitivity of MCH, which was more than that of MCV (97.6% sensitivity) in screening for β-thalassemia carriers. They concluded that the MCH was better than MCH [44].

MCV and MCH are not effective in screening for HbE carriers since mean levels in HbE carriers are just slightly lower than those in normal individuals, but the distribution overlaps substantially. Yeo et al. showed that the use of 80 fL cut-off point could miss cases of HbE carriers [45]. Ittarat et al. showed that 5% of HbE carriers would be missed in 80-fL cut-off points of MCV was used [46]. This group suggested the use of some discriminant functions, F1 = 0.01 × MCH × (MCV) or F2 = RDW × MCH × 2(MCV)/Hb × 100 or F3 = MCV/RBC, to increase effectiveness of using red cell indices for screening for HbE carriers. Our unpublished data showed that using 80-fL and 27 pg cut-off points of MCV and MCH, respectively, did not miss cases HbE carriers regardless of hemoglobin levels (4.2–15.1 g/dL).

2.2 One-tube osmotic fragility test (OFT)

This simple test utilizes osmosis, the movement of water from lower to higher salt concentration region, to test for the osmotic resistance of the red blood cells. In a hypotonic condition, the fixed concentration of salt on the outside is lower than that on the inside of red blood cell, resulting in net water movement into the red blood cell. Normal red blood cells are then lysed and the mixture then turns reddish and clear. Red blood cells of the β-thalassemia and HbE carriers have higher osmotic resistance and thus have slower rupture rate, and the mixture remains turbid. Different laboratories may be using slightly different recipes for preparation of hypotonic salt solution such as 0.36% NaCl in distilled water (DW), 0.36% NaCl in phosphate buffer or buffered saline solution (BSS), and 0.45% NaCl in glycerine or glycerine saline solution (GSS). All of these solutions are normally based on the same concept of kinetic osmotic fragility.

2.2.1 0.36% NaCl-based and BSS-based one-tube osmotic fragility test

By mixing the 20 μL of red blood cells of normal and β-thalassemia carriers in 2 mL of 0.36% NaCl in DW (0.36 g NaCl dissolved in 100 mL DW) or BSS (0.32 g NaCl, 0.05 g Na_2HPO_4, 0.01 g NaH_2PO_4 dissolved in 100 mL DW) and leave for 5 min, the normal red blood cells will completely lyse and the mixture turns

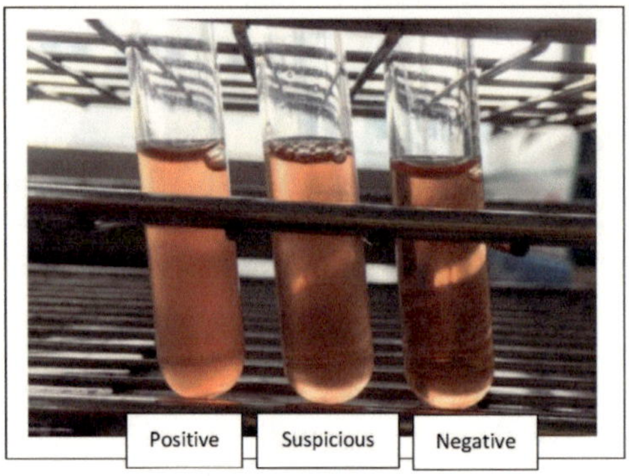

Figure 1.
0.36% NaCl-based and BSS-based one-tube osmotic fragility test for screening of β-thalassemia and HbE carriers. The β-thalassemia carriers all have the positive OFT results, while HbE carriers have either positive, negative, and suspicious OFT results (see the text for detail).

reddish-clear and reported as OFT-Negative. In contrast, the mixture of blood samples of β-thalassemia carriers and 0.36% NaCl remains turbid at 5 min and reported as OFT-Positive. In case that the appearance of the mixture is between positive and negative OFT-results, it is reported as OFT-suspicious (**Figure 1**). Chow et al. showed that this test has 95% sensitivity and 86% specificity for screening the β-thalassemia carrier [47]. Bobhate et al. demonstrated 97.1% sensitivity and 100% specificity of this test, which they called NESTROFT, in screening for β-thalassemia carriers [48], while Mamtani et al. showed 93.4% and 97.2% sensitivity and specificity of this test for screening of the β-thalassemia carriers [49]. For HbE carriers, Fucharoen et al. showed 37.7% false negative OFT result in HbE carriers [50], which was closed to our unpublished data that showed approximately 29.4% false negative results.

2.2.2 0.45% NaCl in glycerine or glycerine saline solution (GSS)-based one-tube osmotic fragility test

This test was established by Prof. Dr. Torpong Sa-nguansermsri of Thalassemia Unit, Department of Pediatrics, Faculty of Medicine, Chiang Mai University and named this test "Erythrocyte Osmotic Fragility Test" (EOFT) [51]. In this platform, the influx of water into the erythrocyte is slow and hemolysis can be measured at any points of time after mixing blood with 0.45% GSS [1.424 g $Na_2HPO_4.2H_2O$, 0.262 g $NaH_2PO_4.2H_2O$, 2.812 g NaCl, 19.27 g glycerine (87%), and DW to make 1000 mL]. Technically, 10 μL of EDTA blood is mixed with 10 mL of 0.45% GSS and read 620-nm absorbance at 15, 30, 45, 60, and 120 s, before calculating hemolysis rate at every time point.

The cut-off point of hemolysis rate is 60%. Positive blood samples have hemolysis rate <60%, while the blood samples having hemolysis rate ≥60% is judged as negative. The β-thalassemia carriers have hemolysis rate of 17.6 ± 8.1%. Hemolysis rate of 32.6 ± 13.2% is observed in HbE carriers [52, 53].

2.2.3 0.45% NaCl in glycerine or glycerine saline solution (GSS)-based one-tube osmotic fragility test expressed in "hemolysis area"

The portable spectrophotometer was invented and capable of reading absorbance and transmission of red light through the red blood cell suspension inside

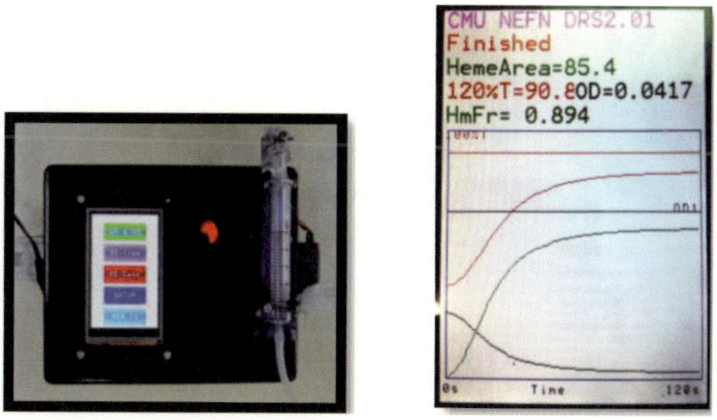

(A) (B)

Figure 2.
Portable spectrophotometer (A) and on-screen GSS-based OFT result with the hemolysis area (HemeArea in the screen) shown in the screen (B).

cuvette [54]. To perform this test, 20 μL of EDTA blood is mixed with 5 mL of GSS in 12 × 75 polypropylene cuvette. Then place the cuvette inside the cuvette holder of the portable spectrophotometer (red dots in **Figure 2(A)**) and start the machine. Light transmission (red line in **Figure 2(B)**), light absorbance (black line in **Figure 2(B)**), and HemeArea or hemolysis area (green line in **Figure 2(B)**) are generated simultaneously in real-time manner. At 120 s, the numeric HemeArea (or hemolysis area) is shown in green alphabets (**Figure 2(B)**).

Cut-off point of the hemolysis area is 52.4 unit. Blood samples having the hemolysis area less than these cut-off values are judged as "positive samples," while those samples having the hemolysis area ≥ 52.4 units are classified as "negative sample." The hemolysis area of normal individuals was 67.1 ± 12.6 units. In contrast, the hemolysis area of HbE carriers, β-thalassemia carriers were found to be 36.4 ± 13.9, 18.6 ± 1.1, respectively [54].

2.3 Dichlorophenolindophenol precipitation (DCIP) test

In dichlorophenolindophenol precipitation (DCIP) test, 2,6-dichiorophenol indophenol (DCIP) were oxidizing chemicals and used as indicator of ascorbic acid measurement. Hemoglobin E is resulted from amino acid change at codon 26 of β-globin chain from glutamic acid to lysine. This change makes contact of α-globin chain and β^E-globin chain less stable. Thus, in DCIP solution, molecule of HbE changes from tetramer to monomer, freeing sulfhydryl group of amino acid, oxidized by the DCIP, denatured, and precipitated [55].

The 500-mL DCIP reagent is composed of 4.36 g Trizma base, 2.68 g EDTA-$Na_2.2H_2O$, 0.0276 g of DCIP, and 0.05 g of saponin. The pH of reagent is adjusted to 7.5 by using 6 N HCl. To perform test, 20 μL of EDTA blood is mixed with 5 mL DCIP reagent. The mixture is incubated in 37°C-water bath for 1 h before precipitation occurs in case of HbE carriers. To enhance visualization, 20 μL of 6% (w/v) ascorbic acid is dropped into the mixture and the color of mixture turns from deep blue to pale red (**Figure 3**).

This test is now commercially available in Thailand. The commercial DCIP reagent has the same ingredient and incubation condition as the original test, except the volume of reagent is scaled down to 2 mL. The examples of commercially DCIP reagent presently distributed in Thailand are THALCON™ and KKU-DCIP™ reagent (**Figure 4**).

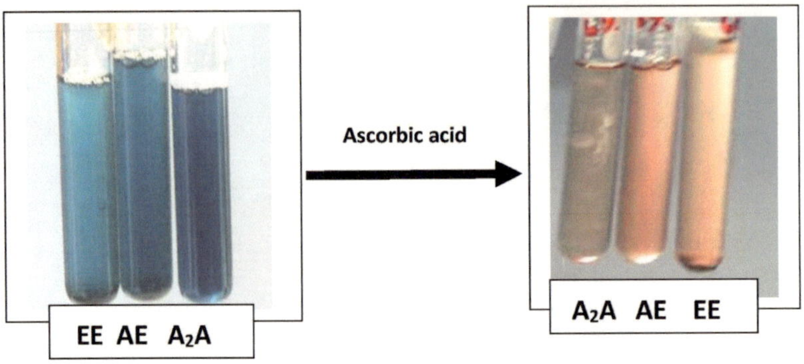

Figure 3.
Dichlorophenolindophenol precipitation (DCIP) test. The DCIP results before adding ascorbic acid have deeply blue color, but after ascorbic acid addition, the color turns to pale red. The amount of precipitation is increased in homozygous HbE (EE), compared to HbE carrier (AE). No precipitation is seen for non-HbE (A_2A). Modified from Ref. [53].

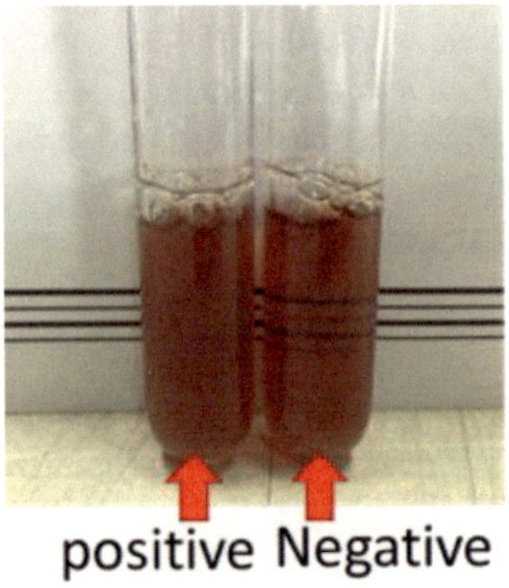

Figure 4.
DCIP test results obtained by commercial DCIP kit. The black lines placed behind the tube aid the result reading. If we cannot see the black lines, the result is positive. If the black lines are clearly seen, the result is negative. DCIP test produces turbid solution.

This test has been validated and shown to be effective in screening for HbE carriers. Analysis in the author's laboratory showed that this test had 100% sensitivity and 98.4% specificity in screening for HbE carriers [56]. Wiwanitkit et al. found almost the same effectiveness of this test in HbE screen; 100% sensitivity and 97.2% specificity [14]. Chapple et al. re-evaluated the KKU-DCIP reagent kit and found 100% sensitivity and 92% specificity for screening for HbE carriers [55].

2.4 HbE-tube test

This test was invented by the author in 2012 [15]. It is based on the principle of anion-exchange liquid chromatography. The diethyl aminoethyl (DEAE)-cellulose having positive charge in buffer having fixed amount of NaCl is placed in the test tube. This condition allows all hemoglobins to bind DEAE-cellulose, except HbE and HbA_2. Then these two hemoglobins will still dissolve in the supernatant. However, since HbE quantity is more than 10% in HbE carriers, then in case of HbE carrier, the supernatant color is red. In contrast, in non HbE, that is, no HbE in blood, the supernatant is colorless (**Figure 5**). This test is simple, requiring no incubation and centrifugation. Standing the test tube after mixing the blood for about 10 min is enough for visualizing the supernatant color.

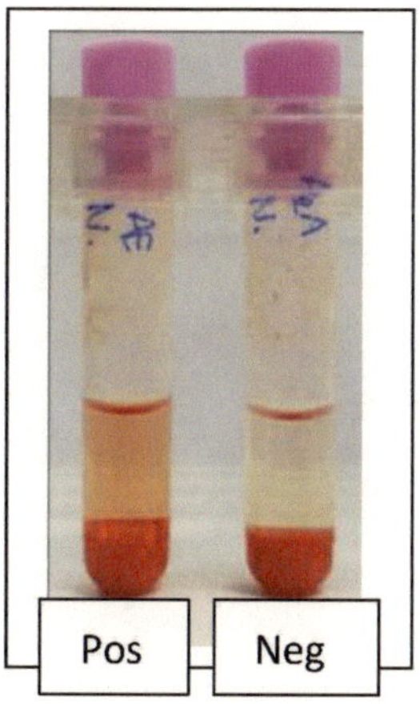

Figure 5.
HbE tube test for screening of HbE carriers. The positive tube (Pos) is the result of HbE carrier having Hb type AE and red supernatant is seen. The negative tube (Neg) is the result of normal individual having Hb type A_2A and colorless supernatant is seen.

To perform the test, 15 μL packed red cell (PRC) is added to pre-prepared DEAE-cellulose suspension in the transparent test tube (0.5 mL DEAE-cellulose suspension in 1.0 mL glycine-NaCl buffer containing 0.2 M glycine–0.01% KCN–7.5 mM NaCl). The tube is shaken briefly, left for 5 min at room temperature, and spun at 3500 round per minute for 5 min before reading the results by visualizing the color of supernatant as shown in **Figure 5**.

This test was simple and effective in screening of HbE carriers. Its sensitivity and specificity for HbE screen are 100%. The reagent can be kept in the cold (2–8°C) for 5 months [15].

2.5 HbE screen test

This test was initially invented by Prof. Dr. Torpong Sa-nguansermsri of The Thalassemia Unit, Department of Pediatrics, Faculty of Medicine, Chiang Mai University, Thailand [57] and adopted for HbE screen in pregnant women by Sirichotiyakul et al. [58]. This test was also established in author's laboratory (Unpublished data). This test works under the principle of anion-exchange column chromatography, modified from microcolumn chromatography for HbA_2 quantification [59, 60].

The test comprises small syringe packed inside with anion-coated resin such as diethylaminoethyl (DEAE)-Sephadex A50 suspended in Tris-HCl-KCN (THK) buffer (6.057 g tris hydroxymethyl aminomethane, 0.1 g KCN, 4 N HCl to adjust pH), pH 8.5. On passing hemolysate through this microcolumn, all hemoglobins bind to the resin. However, passing the eluting buffer (THK buffer, pH 8.2), only HbE and HbA_2 are eluted. If the patients have HbE, the color of entire length of the microcolumn will be red. If the patients do not have HbE, the color of this point will be colorless (**Figure 6**).

To perform this test invented by Prof. Dr. Torpong Sanguansermsri, 10 mL hemoglobin solution (40 μL hemolysate mixed in 5 mL THK buffer pH 8.5) is dropped into microcolumn prepacked with DEAE-Sephadex A 50 to the height of 5.0 cm in pasture pipette. The solution is allowed to flow through the microcolumn which is subsequently equilibrated with 10 mL THK buffer pH 8.5. Finally, HbE and HbA_2 are eluted out of the microcolumn after poring 10 mL of THK buffer, pH 8.2. At the end, the red color of the column is observed. If almost the entire length of microcolumn is red,

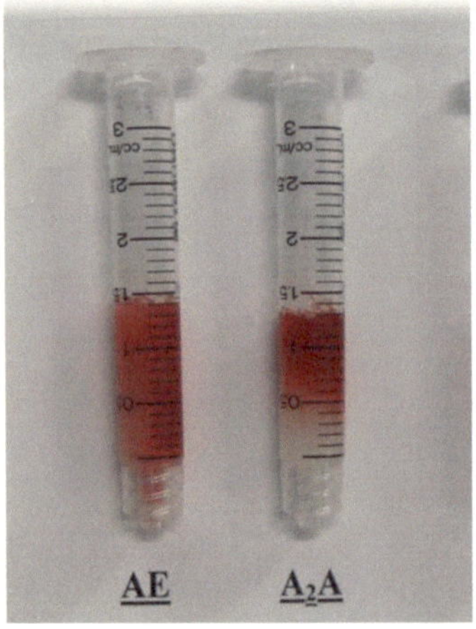

Figure 6.
HbE screening test in a modified protocol so-called naked eye microcolumn for HbE screen (NEMES). The AE sample shows red color in the resin along entire length of the resin, but not for the A_2A sample.

the result is "Positive." However, if the red color sticks to only at the top layer of the packed resin, the result is "Negative" [57]. This test was evaluated by Sirichotiyakul et al. and found to have 100% sensitivity and 100% specificity for HbE screen [58].

Alternatively, the test was modified in author's laboratory. In this modification, DEAE-cellulose was used as the pre-packed resin, and glycine-NaCl buffer was equilibrating and eluting buffer. To prepare microcolumn, DEAE-cellulose resin suspended in equilibrating buffer (0.2 M glycine + 0.01% KCN) is pre-packed to the height of 2.5 cm in 3-mL plastic syringe with 1-cm diameter. To perform the test, 150 μL hemolysate is dropped into the microcolumn and allowed to pass through the resin before eluting HbE with 4 mL eluting buffer (0.2 M glycine + 0.01% KCN + 0.005 M NaCl). The red color of the resin packed in column is observed in the way resemble that mentioned above (**Figure 6**). The protocol was named "Naked-EyE-Microcolumn-HbE-Screen or NEMES" [61]. This test was found to have 100% sensitivity and 100% specificity for screening of HbE carriers.

3. Interpretation of the screening tests

The β-thalassemia carriers always have positive OFT, MCV less than 80 fL, MCH less than 27 pg, and negative HbE. In contrast, HbE carriers may have MCV: more or less than 80 fL, MCH: more or less than 27 pg, OFT: positive or suspicious or negative, and hemolysis area: more or less than 52.4 unit. However, all cases of HbE carriers certainly have positive HbE screening tests performed by all mentioned tests.

The MCV, MCH, and OFT are all positive in β-thalassemia diseases such as homozygous β^O-thalassemia, homozygous β^+-thalassemia, compound heterozygous β^O/β^+-thalassemia, compound heterozygous HbE/β^O-thalassemia, compound heterozygous HbE/β^+-thalassemia, and homozygous HbE. However, the DCIP test, HbE tube test, and HbE screen test are positive in all cases having HbE in blood.

4. Usefulness of screening tests

In financially burden countries that have considerably high prevalence of thalassemia and hemoglobinopathies, initial screen of the carriers in population is essential. This approach helps to decrease the number of cases seeking further for more expensive confirmatory tests. Normally, the sophisticated laboratory tests for conforming the diagnosis of thalassemia and hemoglobinopathies are set up in big centers which are mostly located in the city. Thus, selected cases that are screened in for the definite diagnosis of thalassemia and hemoglobinopathies have to travel a long distance to the city. This would not consume much money for traveling and for laboratory tests.

4.1 Confirmatory method for thalassemia and hemoglobinopathies

Aims of confirmatory tests are to make the definite diagnosis of β-thalassemia and HbE. These tests generally performed only in blood samples having positive results of screening tests. Two sets of confirmatory tests are generally performed; hemoglobin studies and DNA analysis.

4.1.1 Hemoglobin studies by cellulose acetate electrophoresis (CAE) at alkaline condition

This test separates hemoglobins in blood by their negatively molecular net charge. Hemoglobins are allowed to dissolve in Tris-EDTA-Borate (TBE) buffer pH 8.6. This pH is more than isoelectric points (pI) of all hemoglobins (approximately 6.5–7.5) [62, 63]. At this pH, all hemoglobins have negative charge and migrate from cathodic part toward anodic end of the electrophoretic chamber.

In 1 L of TBE buffer, it is composed of 12.0 g tris-hydroxymethyl aminomethane (Tris), 1.22 g ethylenediaminetetraacetic acid (EDTA), and 1.5 g boric acid.

The electrophoresis is performed at a constant voltage of 250–300 volts for 15–20 minutes or until HbA and HbE bands are clearly separated. At the end of electrophoresis, the hemoglobin bands on cellulose acetate plate are stained for 5 minutes with Ponceau S stain (2 g of Ponceau S powder, 30 g of trichloroacetic acid, and 30 g of sulfosalicylic acid in 1 L of distilled water) and destained for 5 minutes in destaining solution (5% acetic acid in distilled water). Finally, the cellulose acetate plate is made clear for permanent record by immersing for 5 minutes in clearing solution (4 volume of methanol +1 volume of glacial acetic acid) and dried by using hair dryer. Hemoglobin pattern from cathodic to anodic ends is Constant Spring-A_2/E/C/O-S/D/Lepore/G-F-A-Portland-Bart's-H [64] (**Figure 7**). Hemoglobin patterns on CAE at alkaline condition are shown in **Table 1**. In the past, densitometer was used to determine quantities of hemoglobins in blood samples. However, this technique is not conventionally performed presently because it may give falsely high levels of hemoglobins if the background is not completely cleared. However, CAE results can still give types of hemoglobins in blood samples. Thus, by

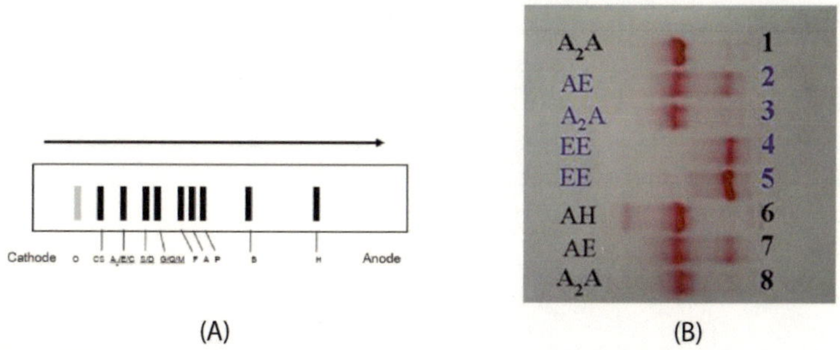

(A) (B)

Figure 7.
(A) Hemoglobin patterns on cellulose acetate electrophoresis (CAE) at pH 8.6. (B) Example of hemoglobin pattern on CAE at pH 8.6 stained with Ponceau S stain.

	Hb patterns on CAE at pH 8.6 of adult
HbE heterozygote (carriers)	EA
HbE homozygote	EE (only 1 band of HbE)
β^O-thalassemia heterozygote (carriers)	A_2A
β^+-thalassemia heterozygote (carriers)	A_2A
β^O-thalassemia homozygote (β^O/β^O)	A_2F
β^+-thalassemia homozygote (β^+/β^+)	A_2FA
β^O/β^+-thalassemia (β^O/β^+)	A_2FA
HbE/β^O-thalassemia (β^E/β^O)	EF
HbE/β^+-thalassemia (β^E/β^+)	EFA

Table 1.
Hemoglobin pattern on CAE at pH 8.6 of β-thalassemia and HbE.

using this technique, further tests must be done in order to determine the level of HbA_2 and HbF. Raised level of HbA_2 beyond normal range is the diagnostic marker for β-thalassemia carriers, while elevated level of HbF helps identify the high HbF condition found in the hereditary persistence of fetal hemoglobin (HPFH).

4.1.2 Hemoglobin study by microcolumn chromatography

This test is preliminarily aimed to quantify HbA_2 levels that help diagnosis of the β-thalassemia carrier. However, HbE has the same pI as HbA_2, thus these two hemoglobins are co-eluted. Microcolumn chromatography is an anion-exchange chromatography-based method. Anion-resin such as DEAE-cellulose or DEAE-Sephadex A50 suspended in appropriate buffer is packed in the microcolumn. On passing hemolysate through the packed resin, negatively charged hemoglobins binds to the resin at different binding affinity. HbA_2 and HbE bind to the resin at the weakest strength (if there is no Hb Constant Spring) and are eluted out easily with small amount of external anion such as CL^-.

There are two types of microcolumn chromatography, based on the anion-resin and buffers used. These include (1) DEAE-Sephadex A50 plus Tris-HCl-KCN buffer, and (2) DEAE-cellulose plus glycine-NaCl buffer.

4.1.2.1 Microcolumn chromatography using DEAE-Sephadex A50 resin

DEAE-Sephadex A 50 resin suspended in Tris-HCl-KCN buffer (0.05 M Tris plus 0.1 g KCN/1 L, adjust pH with 4 N HCl) pH 8.5 is packed in pasture pipette to the height of 8–9 cm [52]. Then, the microcolumn is applied with 100 μL hemolysate, equilibrated with 10 mL THK buffer pH 8.5. Finally, 10 mL THK buffer pH 8.2 is applied to the microcolumn to elute HbA_2 and/or HbE before 10 mL eluate is collected for measuring light absorbance (A) or optical density (OD) at 415 nm. This is then called A_{415}-A_2 or OD_{415}-A_2. For measuring OD_{415} of total hemoglobin or OD_{415}-Total Hb, 100 μL hemolysate is mixed with 10 mL DW before measuring the absorbance. The level of HbA_2 or HbE is calculated by the Eq. 1 shown below.

$$HbA_2 \text{ or } HbE\ (\%) = [OD_{415} - A_2/OD_{415} - \text{total Hb}] \times 100 \quad (1)$$

If percent is less than 10, it is HbA_2.
If percent is 10 up, it is HbE.
Normal range of HbA_2 by this protocol is 2.62 ± 0.87% [52].

4.1.2.2 Microcolumn chromatography using DEAE-cellulose

This protocol was described by Wood [64] and modified in the author's laboratory in 2007 [65].

In modified protocol, DEAE-cellulose resin suspended in equilibrating buffer (0.2 M glycine + 0.01% KCN) is packed to the height of 2 cm in plastic microcolumn with 1.0-cm diameter. Then the microcolumn is applied by 50 μL hemolysate (prepared by mixing 1 part of PRC and 6 parts of 0.05% Triton X-100 as hemolysis buffer) and flushed with 5 mL eluting buffer (0.2 M glycine +0.01% KCN + 0.005 M NaCl). The 5-mL eluate is then collected and measured for absorbance or optical density at 415 nm (A_{415}-A_2 or OD_{415}-A_2). OD_{415} of total hemoglobin is measured in diluted hemolysate (50 μL hemolysate mixed with DW to 15 mL) and called OD_{415}-Total.

Calculation of levels of HbA_2 or HbE must follow the Eq. 2 shown below.

$$HbA_2 \text{ or HbE } (\%) = [OD_{415} - A_2/OD_{415}\text{–total} \times 3] \times 100 \quad (2)$$

If percent is less than 10, it is HbA_2.

If percent is 10 up, it is HbE.

Normal range of HbA_2 by this protocol is 1.3–3.7% (mean 2.5%) [64].

For both protocols, if HbA_2 level is less than 3.5%, the chance of β-thalassemia carrier is excluded. Instead, the cases may be either normal of α-thalassemia carriers. However, if HbA_2 level is between 3.5 and 10.0%, the case is definitely β-thalassemia carrier. In β-thalassemia carriers, mean HbA2 is 4.8% with the range 3.7–7.0% [64].

4.1.2.3 Hemoglobin study by alkaline denaturation test of Betke

This test works under the principle that HbF is resistant to alkaline treatment, while other hemoglobins are not [66]. Therefore, if hemoglobin solution of normal adult is mixed with alkaline solution, HbA, HbA_2 is denatured, leaving only HbF dissolved in the solution. The dissolved HbF can be determined for its level by measuring optical density at 540 nm.

The reagents that are required for this test comprise Drabkin's solution (0.20 g of $K_3Fe(CN)_6$, 0.05 g of KCN, DW to 1 L), 1.2 N NaOH, and saturated ammonium sulphate.

To perform the test, 200 μL hemolysate is mixed in 3.8 mL of Drabkin's solution to prepare cyanmethemoglobin. Thereafter, 2.8 mL of cyanmethemoglobin solution is mixed with 200 μL of 1.2 N NaCl and shaked vigorously for 2 min exactly before adding 2.0 mL of saturated ammonium sulphate. Then, the precipitated hemoglobins are filtered out, and the OD_{540} of filtrate is measured and named OD_{540}-filtrate. OD_{540} of total hemoglobin is measured in a mixture of 400 μL of hemolysate and 6.75 mL of Drabkin's solution and named OD_{540}-Total.

The percentage of HbF is calculated by the following Eq. 3:

$$\text{HbF or Alk F } (\%) = (OD_{540} - \text{filtrate}/OD_{540} - \text{total}) \times 10 \quad (3)$$

Since HbF is determined by alkaline treatment, its level is then named Alkaline F or, simply, Alk F. Besides HbF, Hb Bart's (γ_4) is also resistant to alkaline treatment. This protocol has maximum detection limit at only 50% of HbF. If the alkaline denaturation test is performed in fetal blood sample, the Alk F will not be more than 50%. Therefore, other techniques such as HPLC, CZE should be used to measure HbF in fetal blood.

Alk F is not diagnostic marker for both β-thalassemia carriers and HbE carriers. However, increased HbF level presently is considered advantageous in β-thalassemia and β-hemoglobinopathies [6]. Patients with β-thalassemia disease who also inherit high HbF gene or quantitative trait loci (QTLs) will have mild clinical symptoms. Parents having high HbF gene can pass this gene to their β-thalassemia offspring. Thus, determining HbF in parents is useful in this way.

4.1.2.4 Hemoglobin study by cation-exchange high performance liquid chromatography (HPLC)

Cation-exchange HPLC has become the reference method for typing and quantitating hemoglobins in blood samples [19, 67, 68]. In this system, hemoglobins are dissolved in buffer having a pH of 6.4 that is less than pI of hemoglobins (6.5–7.5) and molecular net charge then is converted to be positive. Different hemoglobins then have different amount of positive charge which determines binding strength of hemoglobins to negatively charged resin. Hb Bart's has the weakest binding affinity, while Hb Constant Spring has the strongest binding affinity. Therefore, on passing external cation, the order of hemoglobins that are eluted fast to slowly should be as follows: Hb Bart's-HbH-HbF-HbAo-HbA2/E-Hb Constant Spring (**Figure 8**).

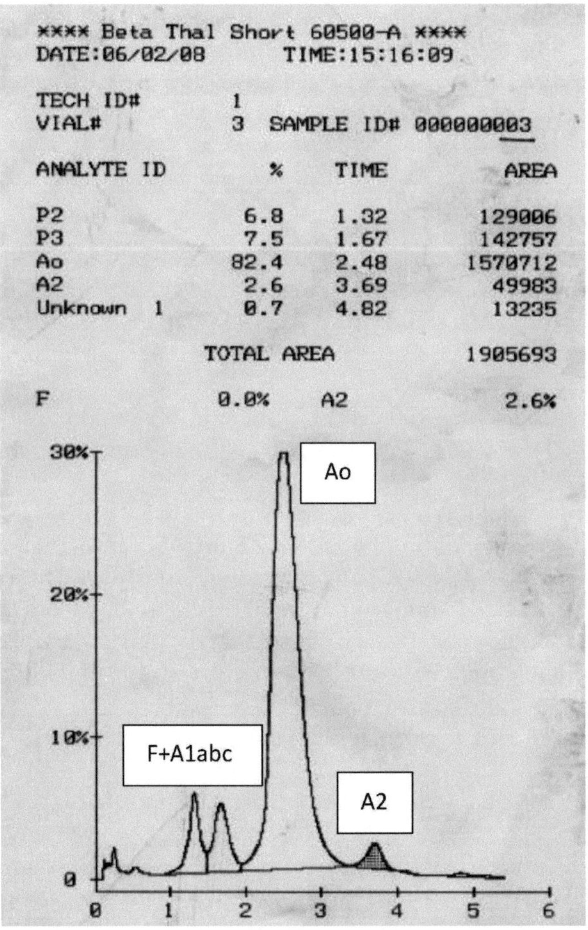

Figure 8.
Hemoglobin pattern of cation-exchange HPLC of normal human adult: A_2A. As shown in the figure, major hemoglobin is HbAo which accounts for 82.4%, while the minor HbA2 accounts for 2.6%. Other minor hemoglobins are labeled P2 and P3, which are Hbs A1a, A1b, and A1c mixture. HbF peak is negligible and reported as 0.0%. This HPLC result may be that of normal individuals or α-thalassemia carriers. It is noted that this kind of cation-exchange HPLC pattern may be also observed in carriers of α-thalassemia 1 and carriers of α-thalassemia 2.

HbA is normally derivatized to several fractions including the minor Hbs A1a, A1b, A1c, and major HbAo. The minor Hbs A1a, A1b, and A1c are eluted just after HbF. For routine Hb typing work, only the major HbAo is usually reported to clinicians. This makes sum of hemoglobin peaks does not equal to 100%.

HbE, which is common in Southeastern part of the world, is co-eluted with HbA_2. However, most of the manufacturers design program to read hemoglobin peak at the A_2 region as only HbA_2. Therefore, the operator must be aware that if the percentage of A_2-peak is more than 10, it is HbE plus HbA_2 and indicates that the sample has HbE. The operator must report HbE or HbE plus HbA_2, instead of reporting HbA_2 as reported by the machine.

There are several manufacturers producing the HPLC machine in the world and the operating procedures as well as quality control protocols are established specifically for each brand. Most importantly, all of these brands generate identical separation peaks of hemoglobins. **Figure 8** shows example of hemoglobin pattern obtained from Variant™ Hemoglobin Analysis System, the widely used HPLC machine in Thailand. In this protocol, the hemoglobin types in normal human adults are A_2A with HbA_2 of 2.6 ± 0.38% [19].

Contrast to the CAE at pH 8.6, hemoglobins separated by the cation-exchange HPLC are automatically calculated for their proportions in blood. Therefore, both types and quantities of hemoglobins are usually obtained when run in this platform.

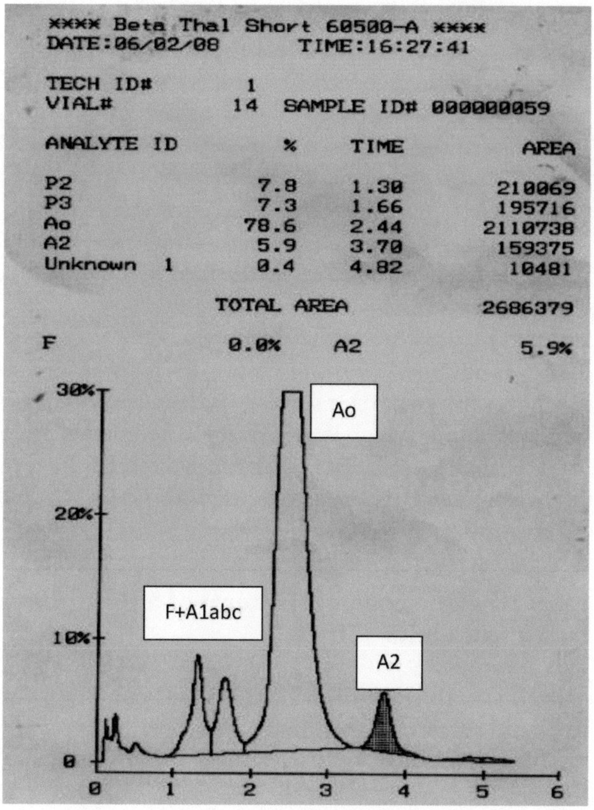

Figure 9.
Hemoglobin pattern of cation-exchange HPLC of β-thalassemia carrier in human adult: A_2A. As shown in the figure, major hemoglobin is HbAo which accounts for 78.6%, while the minor HbA_2 accounts for 5.9%. Other minor hemoglobins are labeled P2 and P3, which are Hbs A1a, A1b, and A1c mixture. HbF peak is negligible and reported as 0.0%.

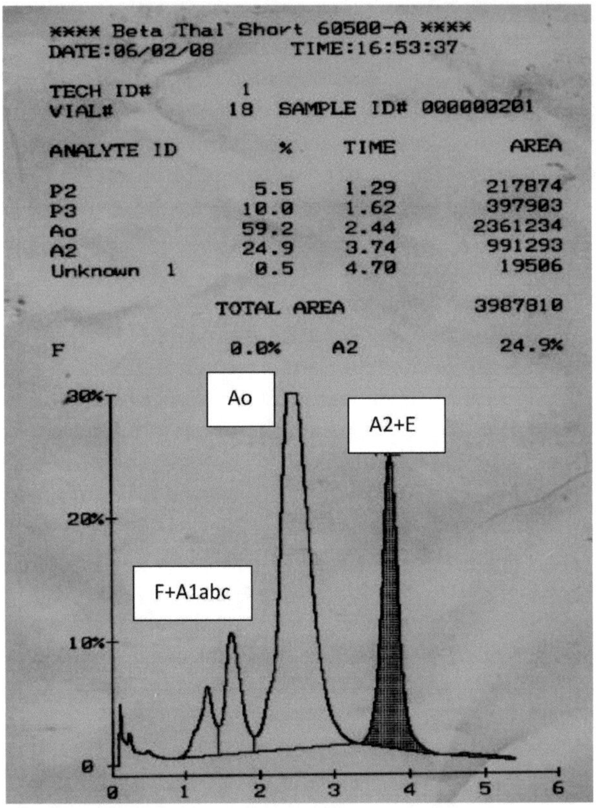

Figure 10.
Hemoglobin pattern of cation-exchange HPLC of HbE carrier in human adults: EA. As shown in the figure, major hemoglobin is HbAo which accounts for 59.2%, while the minor HbE (plus A_2) accounts for 24.9%. Other minor hemoglobins are labeled P2 and P3, which are Hbs A1a, A1b, and A1c mixture. HbF peak is negligible and reported as 0.0%.

4.2 Cation-exchange HPLC hemoglobin patterns of β-thalassemia carriers and HbE carriers in human adults

Hemoglobin patterns obtained from the cation-exchange HPLC of β-thalassemia and HbE are totally different. In carrier state, β-thalassemia carriers in adult life have normal Hb types for adult which is A_2A, but HbA_2 levels is increased to the levels of 5.9 ± 1.35% (**Figure 9**) [19]. HbE carriers in adult life have abnormal Hb typing by the cation-exchange HPLC which is AE with HbE (plus A_2) of 27 ± 3.93% [19], as shown in **Figure 10**.

4.3 Cation-exchange HPLC hemoglobin patterns of β-thalassemia diseases and HbE disease in human adults

Hemoglobin patterns by the cation-exchange HPLC of adult β-thalassemia disease consist of several patterns depending on the combination of the abnormal β-thalassemia mutations.

4.3.1 Homozygous β^O-thalassemia

Individuals of homozygous β^O-thalassemia (β^O/β^O) are usually affected by the severe thalassemia disease and require regular blood transfusion. This group of patients is previously classified as thalassemia major, but now as transfusion dependent thalassemia [69]. Hence, hemoglobin patterns of homozygous β^{O}-thalassemia in adult life of human should consist of HbF and HbA_2 with no HbA prior to blood transfusion, that is, A_2F (**Figure 11**). However, after recent blood transfusion, the hemoglobin types of A_2FA are shown. HbA is certainly from the transfused blood (**Figure 12**).

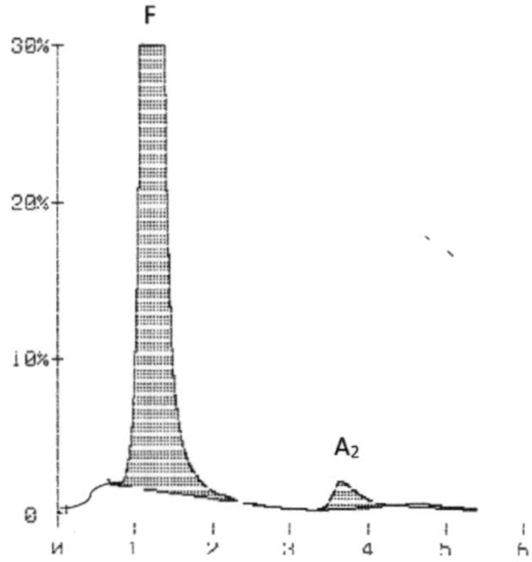

Figure 11.
Cation-exchange HPLC pattern of homozygous β^{O}-thalassemia prior to blood transfusion, which is read as A_2F (F: 97.8%, A_2: 2.2%) (credit to Eaktong Limveeraprajak of Sawan Pracharak Hospital).

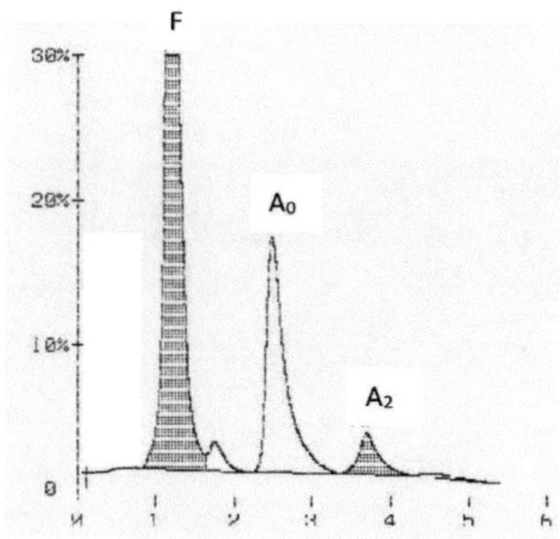

Figure 12.
Cation-exchange HPLC hemoglobin pattern A_2FA seen in homozygous β^{+}-thalassemia and compound heterozygous β^{+}/β^{O}-thalassemia (HbAo: 24.6%, HbF: 68.5%, HbA_2: 3.9%).

4.3.2 Homozygous β^{+}-thalassemia

Individuals of homozygous β^{+}-thalassemia always have mild clinical symptoms and previously are classified as β-thalassemia intermedia. The β-thalassemia intermedia cases usually require no blood transfusion. Thus, now this group of patients is newly classified as non-transfusion dependent thalassemia (NTDT) [69]. Hemoglobin pattern on cation-exchange HPLC of homozygous β^{+}-thalassemia is quite resembling to that of transfused homozygous β^{O}-thalassemia, that is, A_2FA. However, single population of red blood cells on blood smear is also revealed in this homozygous β^{+}-thalassemia, in contrast for dimorphic population in case of transfused homozygous β^{O}-thalassemia. **Figure 12** shows hemoglobin pattern by cation-exchange HPLC of the homozygous β^{+}-thalassemia.

4.3.3 Compound heterozygous β^{O}/β^{+}-thalassemia

Patients with compound heterozygous β^{O}/β^{+}-thalassemia always have severe disease and may require blood transfusion. Thus, they are classified as TDT. Hemoglobin patterns by cation-exchange HPLC of transfused and non-transfused cases is A_2FA, being similar to homozygous β^{+}-thalassemia (**Figure 12**). However, the compound heterozygous β^{O}/β^{+}-thalassemia has thalassemic red blood cell morphology like homozygous β^{O}-thalassemia. In contrast, red blood cell morphology of homozygous β^{+}-thalassemia is less abnormal than the other two β-thalassemia mentioned above.

Hb patterns by the cation-exchange HPLC of adult HbE disease also comprise several varieties depending on combination of β^{E} mutation.

4.3.4 Homozygous HbE

Homozygous HbE (β^{E}/β^{E}) is the mild form of β-thalassemia disease. The patients usually have good clinical symptom with only mild anemia with no need of blood transfusion. Thus, cation-exchange HPLC always shows HbE as major hemoglobin and HbF as the minor hemoglobin; that is, EF (**Figure 13**). Sometime, this hemoglobin type of EF may be confused with that of HbE/β^{O}-thalassemia as HbF in some cases of the later condition may be as low as 4.5% [70] and 2.1% [19]. This low level of HbF may overlap with that seen in homozygous HbE (4.3 ± 2.66%) [19]. Again, red blood cell morphology will help identify if the case is homozygous HbE or the HbE/β^{O}-thalassemia. Red blood cell morphology on

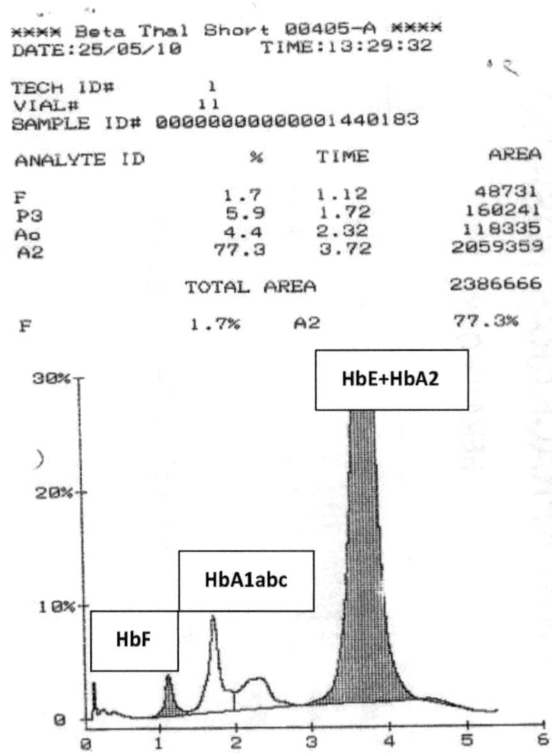

Figure 13.
Hemoglobin pattern by cation-exchange HPLC of homozygous HbE in adults. The major peak contains HbE plus HbA_2, but it is labeled A_2 by software. Thus, level of HbE plus HbA_2 in this case is 77.3, and that of HbF is 1.7%. This case has no HbA, but the software mislabeled the HbA1 fraction as Ao.

blood smear stained with Wright-Giemsa stain is totally different between homozygous HbE and HbE/β^{O}-thalassemia. In homozygous HbE, mild change of red blood cell morphology with considerable amount of target cells is usually observed. In contrast, thalassemia type of red blood cell morphology is typical for the HbE/β^{O}-thalassemia.

4.3.5 Compound heterozygous β^{E} and β^{O}-thalassemia

Individuals with compound heterozygote of β^{E} and β^{O}-thalassemia are always affected by the thalassemia disease and some require blood transfusion. Therefore, the hemoglobin patterns by cation-exchange HPLC of this case will be EF (61.2 ± 13.6% HbE, 31.1 ± 14.5% HbF) prior to blood transfusion [19] and EFA after recent blood transfusion (**Figure 14**).

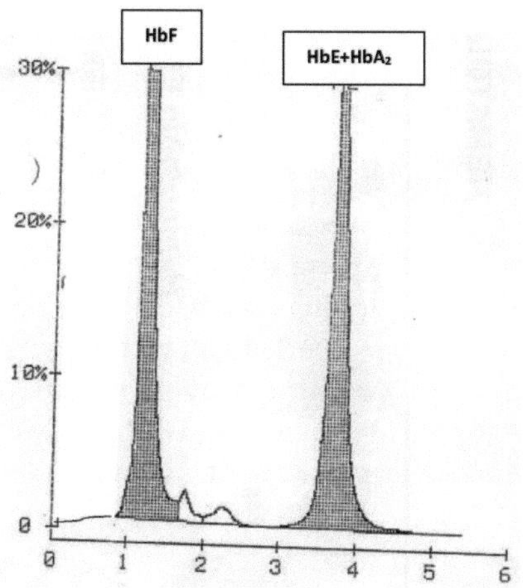

Figure 14.
Hemoglobin pattern in cation-exchange HPLC of cases with HbE/β^{O}-thalassemia (F 53.1%, E 35.8%).

4.3.6 Compound heterozygous β^{E} and β^{+}-thalassemia

Individuals with compound heterozygote of β^{E} and β^{+}-thalassemia have mild clinical symptoms and classified as NTDT. Therefore, interference of transfused blood is not possible. The cation-exchange HPLC pattern of hemoglobin in this case should be EFA. This is because some β-globin chains are still produced.

4.3.7 Double form of HbE carrier and HbH disease

This thalassemia syndrome is conventionally termed AEBart's disease. This is a mild form of α-thalassemia syndrome, and blood transfusion is not required. Thus, transfused blood would not also interfere result reading in this situation. Hemoglobins A, E (with A_2), Bart's are always seen under the cation-exchange HPLC (**Figure 15**). This is why it is called AEBart's disease.

4.3.8 Double form of HbE homozygote and HbH disease

This is also a mild form of α-thalassemia disease that shows hemoglobins E, F, and Bart's in the cation-exchange HPLC. It is thus called EFBart's disease. By running the cation-exchange HPLC, Hbs E, F, and Bart's are always seen in the chromatogram.

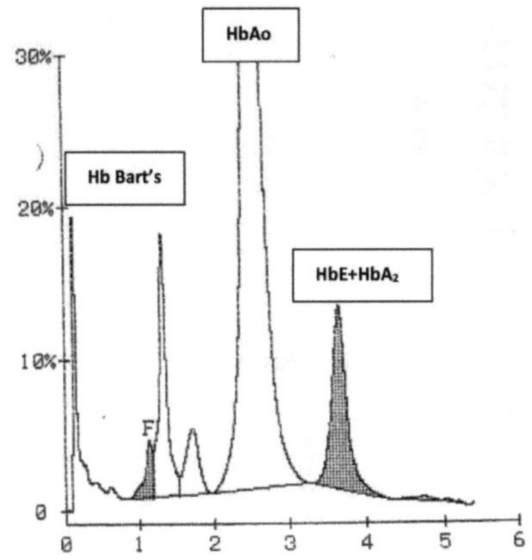

Figure 15.
Cation-exchange HPLC of hemoglobin component in AEBart's disease. HbE: 13.5%, HbA_0: 71.8%, Hb Bart's (no numeric proportion as the analysis software was not designed for Hb Bart's quantification).

4.3.9 Double form of HbE/β^O-thalassemia and HbH disease

This is a rare form of thalassemia syndrome. On running in the cation-exchange HPLC, EFBart's pattern of hemoglobin is also seen, being similar to the double form of homozygous HbE and HbH disease. Red blood cell morphology on blood smear may help differentiate these two conditions, but skillful personnels are needed to examine red blood cell morphology. However, DNA analysis in the only technique that can correctly differentiate this EFBart's syndrome.

5. Hemoglobin study by capillary zone electrophoresis (CZE)

Capillary zone electrophoresis (CZE) has been introduced for use as a tool for analysis of hemoglobin variants [23–27, 71]. Conventionally, separation of hemoglobin is performed in alkaline condition, in which HbH has the maximum molecular negative charge, followed, respectively, by Hb Bart's, HbA, HbF, $HbsA_2$/E, and Hb Constant Spring. The separation is based on high voltage (7500 V) and electro-endo-osmotic force (EOF). Hemoglobins are forced in the system to move from anode to cathode with the cuvette placed at the cathodic end. Once hemoglobin band moves into the cuvette, the 415-nm absorbance is measured and the light signals are converted by the software to electropherogram. Each hemoglobin has its own location or zone in the electropherogram, HbCS-zone 2: Z(C), HbA_2-zone 3: Z(A_2), HbE-zone 4: Z(E), HbF-zone 7: Z(F), HbA-zone 9: Z (A), Hb Bart's – zone 12, and Hb H – zone 15. HbE and HbA_2 are clearly separated by this system (**Figures 16** and **17**).

5.1 The CZE pattern of β-thalassemia carriers and HbE carriers

In β-thalassemia carrier at adult life, the CZE pattern of hemoglobin is similar to that obtained from cation-exchange HPLC. The normal hemoglobin typing result of A_2A or A_2FA with HbA_2 levels of more than 3.5% (5.4 ± 0.5%) and HbF levels of less than 2% (0.9 ± 1.4%) are always observed [27] (**Figure 18**).

In HbE carrier of adult life, the hemoglobin pattern of CZE is different from that of cation-exchange HPLC. HbE and HbA_2 co-eluted in the cation-exchange HPLC. In CZE, HbE moves behind HbA_2. Thus, hemoglobin pattern of HbE carrier

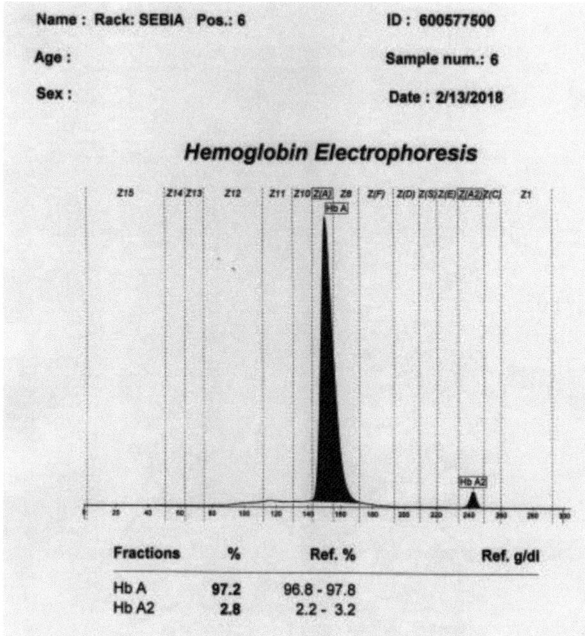

Figure 16.
CZE electropherogram of normal human hemoglobins. HbA: 94.3%, HbF: 2.4%, HbA$_2$: 3.3%.

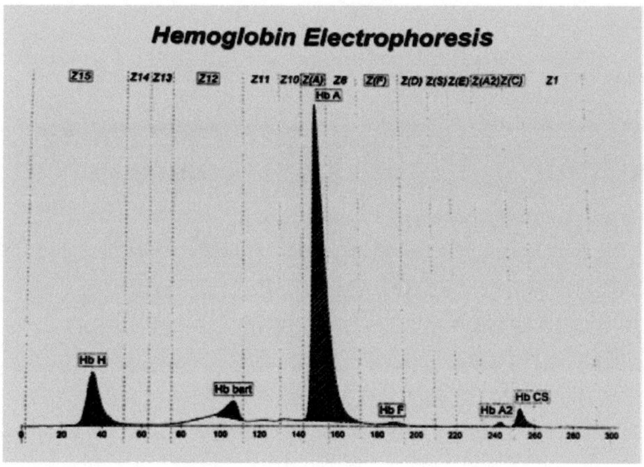

Figure 17.
CZE pattern of hemoglobins from zone (Z) 1 to zone (Z) 15.

in CZE should be A$_2$EFA. The percentage of these hemoglobins is as follows: HbA$_2$: 3.5 ± 0.4%, HbE: 25.6 ± 1.4%, and HbF: 0.4 ± 0.8% [27]. HbE level in the CZE system is usually lower than that obtained from cation-exchange HPLC (27.8 ± 7.5%). This is due to the fact that the level of HbE from HPLC is the sum of HbE and HbA$_2$ that are co-eluted, while only HbE is reported in the CZE system. Thus, performers must be careful in reporting HbE. HbA$_2$ level is slightly elevated. This confirms that HbE carrier also acts as mild β-thalassemia carrier (**Figure 19**).

5.2 The CZE pattern in β-thalassemia disease and HbE disease

CZE pattern of hemoglobins in β-thalassemia disease in adults depends on types of the disease. Although, principles of separation are different, the patterns of hemoglobin

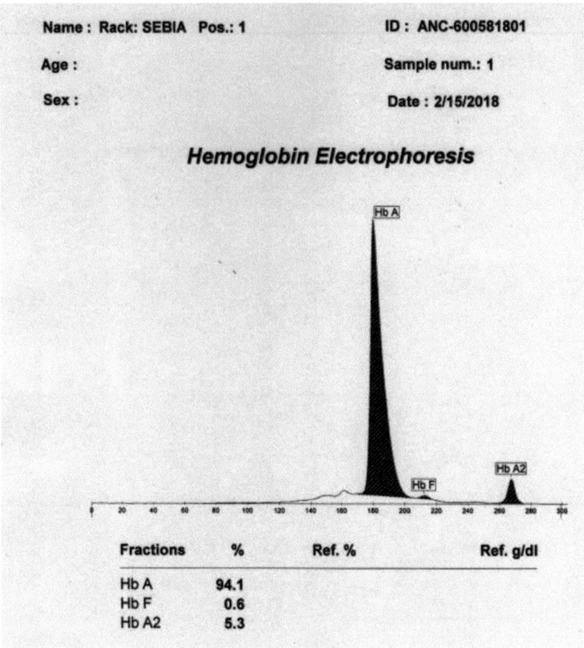

Figure 18.
CZE pattern of hemoglobins of β-thalassemia carrier.

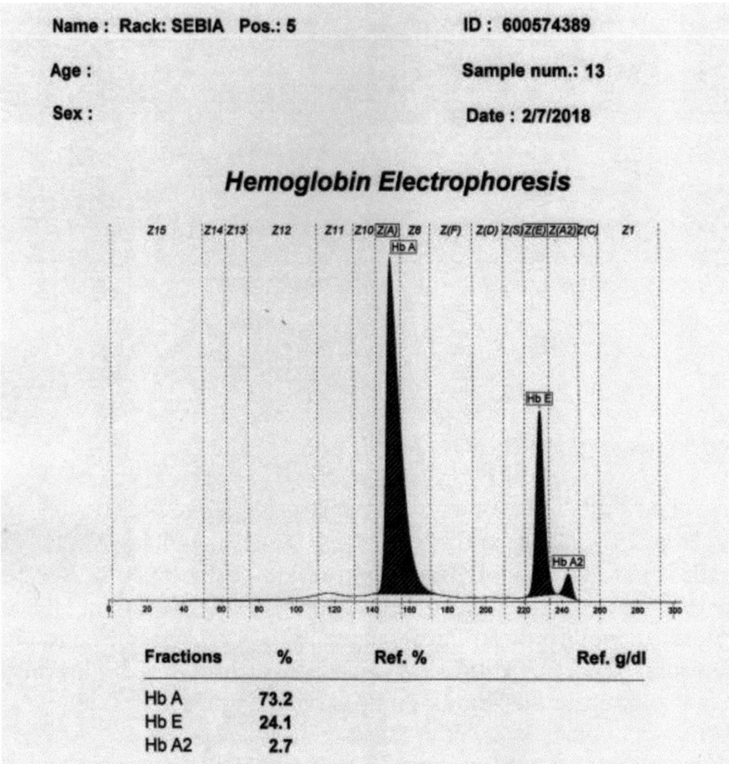

Figure 19.
CZE pattern of hemoglobin of HbE carrier.

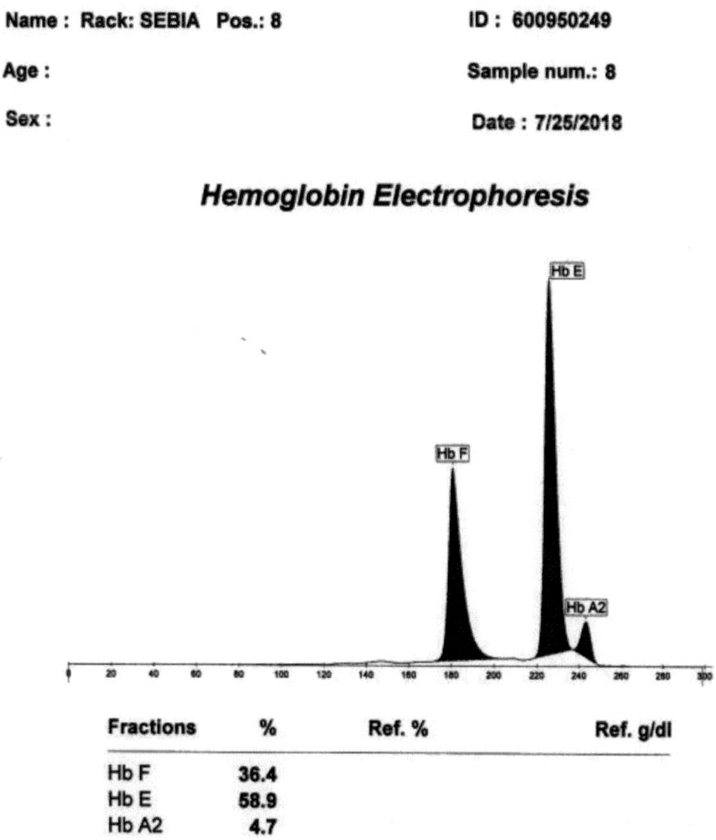

Figure 20.
CZE pattern of hemoglobins of HbE/β^O-thalassemia, composing of A_2EF with 4.7% HbA2, 58.9% HbE, and 36.4% HbF.

in β-thalassemia disease and HbE disease obtained from CZE are quite similar to those obtained from cation-exchange HPLC. For homozygous β^O-thalassemia, A_2F is the typical hemoglobin typing results. For homozygous β^+-thalassemia and compound heterozygous β^+/β^O-thalassemia, the A_2FA is generally seen in CZE platform.

CZE patterns of hemoglobins in HbE disease in adults also depend on types of the diseases. However, as HbE and HbA_2 are clearly separated in the CZE platform, these two hemoglobins must be separately reported. For example, in HbE/β^O-thalassemia, for example, A_2EF must be reported together with the proportion of each hemoglobin (**Figure 20**).

6. Hemoglobin study by monoclonal antibody

Thalassemia and hemoglobinopathies can be identified accurately by using monoclonal antibodies (mAbs) against human hemoglobins [72, 73]. Application of mAb-based protocols aims primarily to identify the carriers of thalassemia and hemoglobinopathies. For instance, α-thalassemia carrier can be detected by using mAbs against Hb Bart's [29] and HbH [74]. Immunochromatographic strip test utilizing mAb to Hb Bart's was produced and successfully applied for screening α-thalassemia carriers [32, 75].

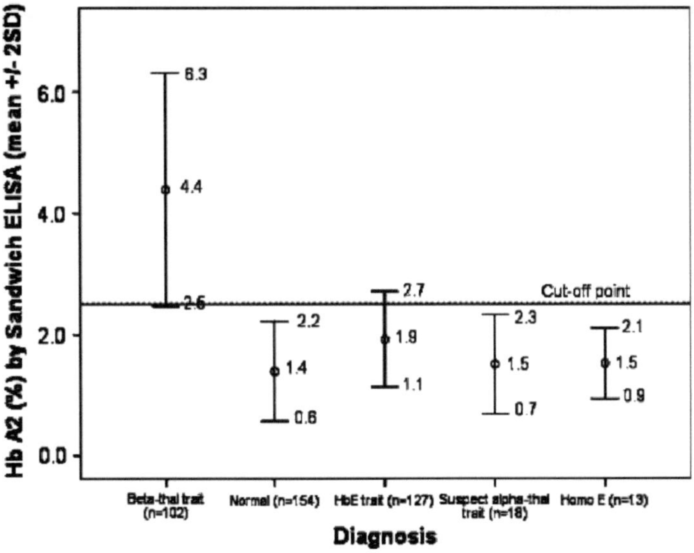

Figure 21.
HbA_2 levels determined by sandwich ELISA set up in the author's laboratory. Note that HbA_2 levels in β-thalassemia trait are higher than those in normal, HbE trait, homozygous HbE, and suspected α-thalassemia trait (modified from [30]).

The β-thalassemia carrier can also be identified by using antigen-antibody reaction. Since elevated HbA_2 level has been shown to be diagnostic marker of the β-thalassemia carrier, mAbs against δ-globin chain of HbA_2 were produced and ELISA set up to quantify HbA_2 levels by Shyamala et al. [76]. Using this ELISA, Shyamala found mean value of HbA_2 in normal and β-thalassemia carrier to be 2.5 and 5.4%, respectively. The mAb against HbA_2 was also produced and sandwich ELISA developed in the author's laboratory [30]. Under this developed sandwich ELISA, Kuntaruk found that the levels of HbA_2 between normal and β-thalassemia carrier were also significantly different (**Figure 21**). Thus, the β-thalassemia carrier can be identified by the sandwich ELISA to quantify HbA_2 level.

7. DNA analysis for β-thalassemia and HbE

Analysis of mutations in β-globin gene to identify β-thalassemia and HbE is now performed routinely in most laboratories. The finding of the causative point mutations in the β-globin gene provides definite diagnosis of these disorders. More than 900 point mutations have been reported for β-thalassemia and β-hemoglobinopathies (Globin Gene Server: http://globin.cse.psu.edu/). Certain ethic groups have their own pattern of point mutations of β-globin gene [2, 4, 77, 78].

There are several allele-specific PCR protocols for detecting both carrier and disease state of β-thalassemia and HbE. These include mutagenically separated (MS)-PCR [35] and amplification refractory mutation system (ARMS)-PCR [79]. These two protocols were modified and adapted in author's laboratory. Another allele-specific PCR protocol was established in the author's laboratory and named "Multiplex Allele-Specific (MAS)-PCR" [29].

7.1 Identification of β-thalassemia and HbE by MS-PCR

The MS-PCR was used to detect β-globin gene mutations by several centers. In author's laboratory, this PCR protocol was modified and adapted to identify the β-globin gene mutations commonly found in Thai individuals. These included TTCT deletion or 4 bp-deletion at codons 41/42 ($\beta^{41/42}$) and A > T substitution at codon 17 (β^{17}) of β-globin gene [80]. These two mutations have been shown to account for approximately 67.5% in Thais by author's survey [29] and 83.9% by others' studies [81]. The MS-PCR was performed in the author's laboratory under the protocol described previously.

7.1.1 MS-PCR for $\beta^{41/42}$ mutation

Procedure: The 25-μL PCR is performed containing 250 ng genomic DNA, 200 μM of each dNTP; 0.5 units Taq DNA polymerase, 100 ng of "Common primer" for $\beta^{41/42}$; 5′-TCA TTC GTC TGT CCA TTC TAA AC-3′, 150 ng of "Normal primer" for $\beta^{41/42}$; 5′-TTC CCA CCA TTA GGC TGC TGG TGG TCT ACC CTT GGA CCC AGA GGT TCT T-3′, 250 ng of "Mutant primer" for $\beta^{41/42}$; 5′-ACC CTT GGA CCC AGA GGT TGA G-3′, 10 mM Tris pH 8.8; 50 mM KCl and 1.5 mM of $MgCl_2$.

Thermal cycles: A total of 35 thermal cycles was carried out with each cycle comprising DNA denaturation at 94°C for 1 min, primer annealing at 56°C for 1 min, and primer extension at 72°C for 1 min; the initial denaturation was extended to 4 min while the final extension was prolonged to 5 min.

Detection of amplified products: The amplified products were separated in 2.5% agarose gel electrophoresis at 120 V for 15–20 min before visualizing with a UV-transilluminator. The fragments sizing 324 and 351 bp indicate presence and absence of the $\beta^{41/42}$ mutation, respectively (**Figure 22**).

Interpretation: Samples having only 324-bp amplified fragments are homozygote for $\beta^{41/42}$ with genotype $\beta^{41/42}/\beta^{41/42}$. Samples having only 351-bp fragments are negative for the $\beta^{41/42}$ with genotype β^A/β^A or β^T/β^T (A represents HbA; T represents other types of β-globin gene mutation). Samples having both 324 and 351-bp amplified products are heterozygote for the $\beta^{41/42}$ with genotype of either $\beta^{41/42}/\beta^A$ or $\beta^{41/42}/\beta^T$ (A represents HbA; T represents other types of β-globin gene mutation).

7.1.2 MS-PCR for β^{17} mutation

Procedure: The 25-μL PCR is performed containing 250 ng genomic DNA, 200 μM of each dNTP; 0.5 units Taq DNA polymerase, 100 ng of "Common primer" for β^{17}; 5′-GGC AGA GAG AGT CAG TGC CTA-3′, 150 ng of "Normal

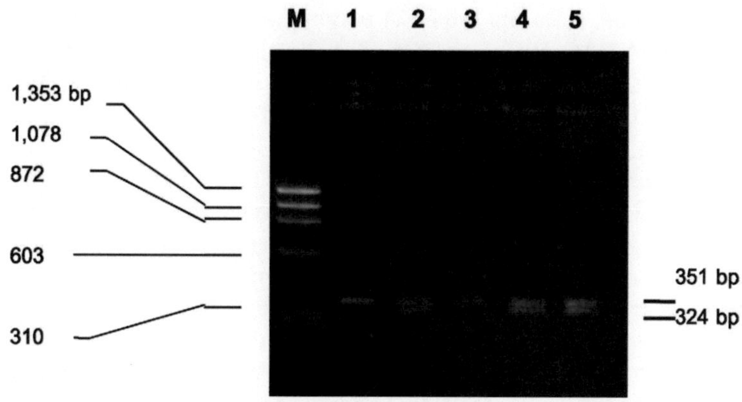

Figure 22.
MS-PCR for detecting $\beta^{41/42}$ mutation. Lanes 1 and 3 are negative for the $\beta^{41/42}$ mutations as only 351-bp amplified products are seen. Lanes 2, 4, and 5 are heterozygote for the $\beta^{41/42}$ mutation as both 3510 and 324-bp amplified products are seen.

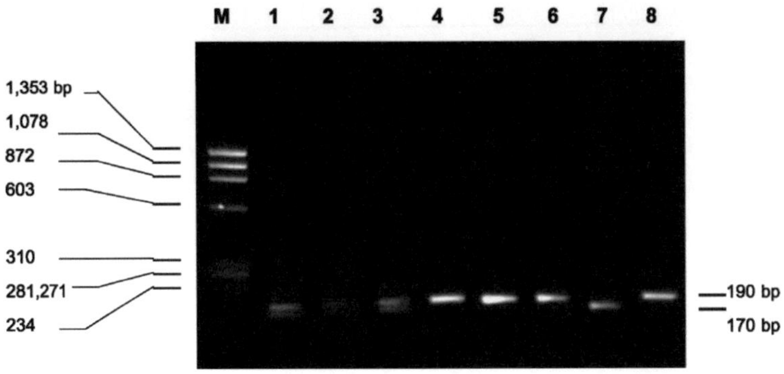

Figure 23.
MS-PCR for identifying β^{17} mutation. Lanes 4, 5, 6, and 8 are negative for the β^{17} mutation as only 190-bp amplified products are seen. Lanes 7 is homozygote for the β^{17} mutation as only 170-bp amplified products is seen. Lanes 1, 2, and 3 are heterozygote for the β^{17} mutation since both 170 and 190-bp amplified products are seen.

primer" for β^{17}; 5′-ACC TGA CTC CTG AGG AGA AGA CTG CCG TTA CTG CCC TGT GGG ACA-3′, 100 ng of "Mutant primer" for β^{17}; 5′-TCT GCC GTT ACT GCC CTG TGG CAC-3′, 10 mM Tris pH 8.8; 50 mM KCl and 1.5 mM of $MgCl_2$.

Thermal cycles: A total of 35 thermal cycles was carried out with each cycle comprising DNA denaturation at 94°C for 1 min, primer annealing at 59°C for 1 min, and primer extension at 72°C for 1 min; the initial denaturation was extended to 4 min while the final extension was prolonged to 5 min.

Detection of amplified products: The amplified products were separated in 2.5% agarose gel electrophoresis at 120 V for 15–20 min before visualizing with a UV-transilluminator. The fragments sizing 170 and 190 bp indicate presence and absence of the β^{17} mutation, respectively (**Figure 23**).

Interpretation: Samples having only 170-bp amplified fragments are homozygote for β^{17} with genotype β^{17}/β^{17}. Samples having only 190-bp fragments are negative for the β^{17} with genotype β^{A}/β^{A} or β^{T}/β^{T} (A represents HbA; T represents other types of β-globin gene mutation). Samples having both 170 and 190-bp amplified products are heterozygote for the β^{17} with genotype of either β^{17}/β^{A} or β^{17}/β^{T} (A represents HbA; T represents other types of β-globin gene mutation).

7.1.3 MS-PCR for β^{E} mutation or HbE

Procedure: The 25-μL PCR is performed containing 250 ng genomic DNA, 200 μM of each dNTP; 0.5 units Taq DNA polymerase, 100 ng of "Common primer" for β^{E}; 5′-GGC AGA GAG AGT CAG TGC CTA-3′, 100 ng of "Normal primer" for β^{E}; 5′-CGT GGA TGA AGT TGG TGG AG-3′, 150 ng of "Mutant primer" for β^{E}; 5′-CTG CCC TGT GGG CAA GGT GAA CGT GGA TGA AGT TGG TGG AA-3′, 10 mM Tris pH 8.8; 50 mM KCl and 1.25 mM of $MgCl_2$.

Thermal cycles: A total of 35 thermal cycles was carried out with each cycle comprising DNA denaturation at 94°C for 1 min, primer annealing at 56°C for 1 min and primer extension at 72°C for 1 min; the initial denaturation was extended to 4 min while the final extension was prolonged to 5 min.

Detection of amplified products: The amplified products were separated in 2.5% agarose gel electrophoresis at 120 V for 15–20 min before visualizing with a UV-transilluminator. The fragments sizing 160 and 138 bp indicate presence and absence of the β^{E} mutation, respectively (**Figure 24**).

Interpretation: Samples having only 160-bp amplified fragments are homozygote for β^{E} with genotype β^{E}/β^{E}. Samples having only 138-bp fragments are negative for the β^{E} with genotype β^{A}/β^{A} or β^{T}/β^{T} (A represents HbA; T represents other types

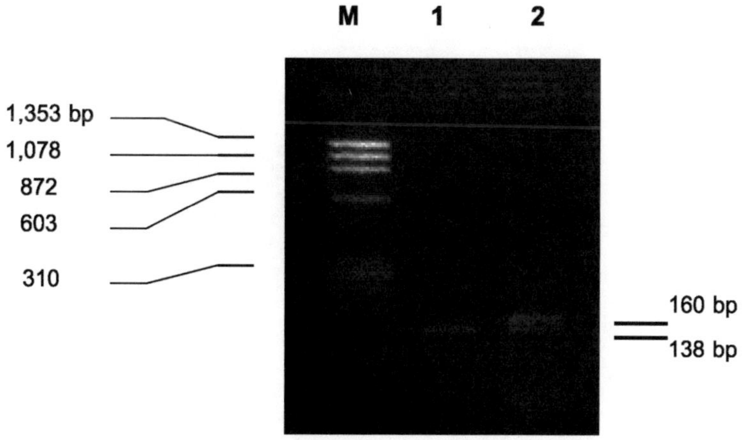

Figure 24.
MS-PCR for identifying β^E mutation. Lane 1 is negative for the βE mutation as only 138-bp amplified products is seen. Lane 2 is heterozygote for βE mutation as both 138-bp and 160-bp amplified products are seen.

of β-globin gene mutation). Samples having both 138 and 160-bp amplified products are heterozygote for the β^E with genotype of either β^E/β^A or β^E/β^T (A represents HbA; T represents other types of β-globin gene mutation).

8. Identification of β-thalassemia and HbE by ARMS-PCR

ARMS-PCR was established by Old et al. [79]. This technique also uses three oligonucleotide primers. However, the length of normal and mutant primers is similar. Therefore, size of normal and mutant amplified products is the same and cannot be separated in the agarose gel electrophoresis. Thus, two PCRs must be performed in the ARMS-PCR. Both PCRs have the same ingredients, except normal and mutant oligonucleotide primers are added in separated reaction tubes (M and N-tube). In addition, a pair of oligonucleotide primers specific to other gene must also be added into both PCRs. The amplified products obtained by this pair of primers are the internal control for the ARMS-PCR.

8.1 ARMS-PCR for $\beta^{41/42}$

Procedure: Two 25-μL reactions are performed; M-reaction and N-reaction. Both M and N-reactions contain 150 ng genomic DNA, 200 μM of each dNTP; 0.6 units Taq DNA polymerase, 0.2 μM of "S-primer"; 5′-ACC TCA CCC TGT GGA GCC AC-3′, 0.15 μM of "M41/42 primer"; 5′-GAG TGG ACA GAT CCC CAA AGG ACT CAA CCT–3′ (for M-reaction only), 0.15 μM of "N41/42 primer"; 5′-GAG TGG ACA GAT CCC CAA AGG ACT CAA AGA-3′ (for N-reaction only), 0.2 μM of "P1 primer"; 5′-GCG ATC TGG GCT CTG TGT TCT-3′, 0.2 μM of "P2 primer"; 5′-GTT CCC TGA GCC CCG ACA CG-3′, 10 mM Tris pH 8.8; 50 mM KCl and 1.5 mM of $MgCl_2$.

Thermal cycles: A total of 35 thermal cycles was carried out with each cycle comprising DNA denaturation at 95°C for 1 min, primer annealing at 65°C for 1 min and primer extension at 72°C for 1 min; the initial denaturation was extended to 5 min while the final extension was prolonged to 5 min.

Detection of amplified products: The amplified products were separated in 2.5% agarose gel electrophoresis at 120 V for 15–20 min before visualizing with a UV-transilluminator. The fragments sizing 439 bp is the specific amplified products, and the PCR products sizing 314 bp are the control products (**Figure 25**).

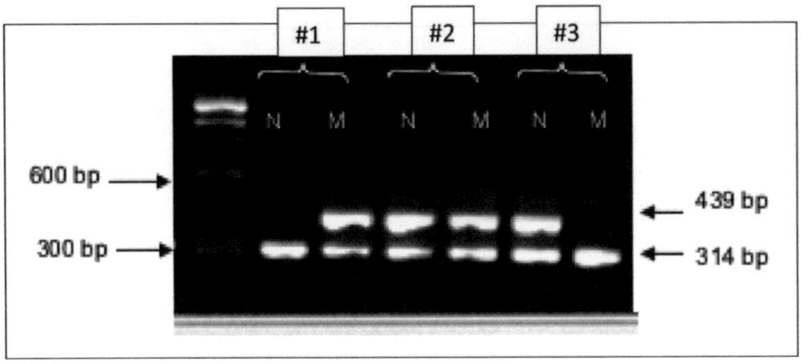

Figure 25.
ARMS-PCR for identifying the $\beta^{41/42}$ mutation. The 314-bp amplified products are internal control. The 439-bp amplified products are the $\beta^{41/42}$ specific products. Sample #1 is homozygote for $\beta^{41/42}$ mutation as the 439-pb amplified products are seen in only "M-reaction." Sample #3 is negative for the $\beta^{41/42}$ mutation since the 439-bp amplified products are seen in only "N-reaction." Sample #2 is heterozygote for the $\beta^{41/42}$ mutation since the 439-bp amplified products are seen in both "M-reaction" and "N-reaction."

Interpretation: Both M and N-reactions must have the 314-bp control products and the results can be read. It both M and N-reactions have 439-bp PCR products, the samples are heterozygote for $\beta^{41/42}$ with genotype of either $\beta^{41/42}/\beta^{A}$ or $\beta^{41/42}/\beta^{T}$ (A represents HbA; T represents other types of β-globin gene mutation). If the 439-bp PCR products are seen in only M-reaction, the samples are homozygote for $\beta^{41/42}$ with genotype $\beta^{41/42}/\beta^{41/42}$. If samples have the 439-bp PCR products in only N-reaction, the samples are negative for the $\beta^{41/42}$ with genotypes of either β^{A}/β^{A} or β^{T}/β^{T} (A represents HbA; T represents other types of β-globin gene mutation) (**Figure 25**).

8.2 ARMS-PCR for β17

Procedure: Two 25-μL reactions are performed; M-reaction and N-reaction. Both M and N-reactions contain 150 ng genomic DNA, 200 μM of each dNTP; 0.6 units Taq DNA polymerase, 0.2 μM of "S-primer"; 5′-ACC TCA CCC TGT GGA GCC AC-3′, 0.15 μM of "M17 primer"; 5′-CTC ACC ACC AAC TCA GCC ACG TTC AGC ATA-3′ (for M-reaction only), 0.15 μM of "N17 primer"; 5′-CTC ACC ACC AAC TTC ATC CAC GTT CAC ATT-3′ (for N-reaction only), 0.2 μM of "P1 primer"; 5′-GCG ATC TGG GCT CTG TGT TCT-3′, 0.2 μM of "P2 primer"; 5′-GTT CCC TGA GCC CCG ACA CG-3′, 10 mM Tris pH 8.8; 50 mM KCl and 1.5 mM of $MgCl_2$.

Thermal cycles: A total of 35 thermal cycles was carried out with each cycle comprising DNA denaturation at 95°C for 1 min, primer annealing at 65°C for 1 min and primer extension at 72°C for 1 min; the initial denaturation was extended to 5 min while the final extension was prolonged to 5 min.

Detection of amplified products: The amplified products were separated in 2.5% agarose gel electrophoresis at 120 V for 15–20 min before visualizing with a UV-transilluminator. The fragments sizing 239 bp is the specific amplified products, and the PCR products sizing 314 bp are the control products (**Figure 26**).

Interpretation: Both M and N-reactions must have the 314-bp control products and the results can be read. If both M- and N-reactions have 239-bp PCR products, the samples are heterozygote for β^{17} with genotype of either β^{17}/β^{A} or β^{17}/β^{T} (A represents HbA; T represents other types of β-globin gene mutation). If the 239-bp PCR products are seen in only M-reaction, the samples are homozygote for β^{17} with genotype β^{17}/β^{17}. If samples have the 239-bp PCR products in only N-reaction, the samples are negative for the β^{17} with genotypes of either β^{A}/β^{A} or β^{T}/β^{T} (A represents HbA; T represents other types of β-globin gene mutation) (**Figure 26**).

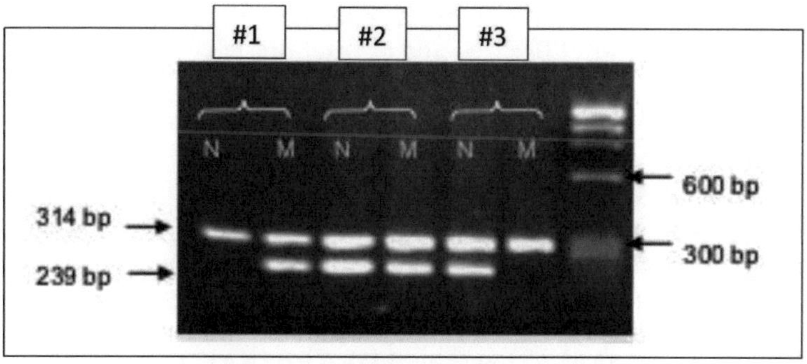

Figure 26.
ARMS-PCR for identifying the β^{17} mutation. The 314-bp amplified products are internal control. The 239-bp amplified products are the β^{17} specific products. Sample #1 is homozygote for β^{17} mutation as the 239-pb amplified products are seen in only "M-reaction." Sample #3 is negative for the β^{17} mutation since the 239-bp amplified products are seen in only "N-reaction." Sample #2 is heterozygote for the β^{17} mutation since the 239-bp amplified products are seen in both "M-reaction" and "N-reaction."

8.3 ARMS-PCR for β^E

Procedure: Two 25-μL reactions are performed; M-reaction and N-reaction. Both M and N-reactions contain 150 ng genomic DNA, 200 μM of each dNTP; 0.6 units Taq DNA polymerase, 0.2 μM of "S-primer"; 5′-ACC TCA CCC TGT GGA GCC AC-3′, 0.15 μM of "HbE-M primer"; 5′-TAA CCT TGA TAC CAA CCT GCC CAG GGC GTT-3′ (for M-reaction only), 0.15 μM of "HbE-N primer"; 5′-TAA CCT TGA TAC CAA CCT GCC CAG GGC GTC-3′ (for N-reaction only), 0.2 μM of "P1 primer"; 5′-GCG ATC TGG GCT CTG TGT TCT-3′, 0.2 μM of "P2 primer"; 5′-GTT CCC TGA GCC CCG ACA CG-3′, 10 mM Tris pH 8.8; 50 mM KCl and 1.5 mM of $MgCl_2$.

Thermal cycles: A total of 35 thermal cycles was carried out with each cycle comprising DNA denaturation at 95°C for 1 min, primer annealing at 65°C for 1 min and primer extension at 72°C for 1 min; the initial denaturation was extended to 5 min while the final extension was prolonged to 5 min.

Detection of amplified products: The amplified products were separated in 2.5% agarose gel electrophoresis at 120 V for 15–20 min before visualizing with a UV-transilluminator. The fragments sizing 260 bp is the specific amplified products, and the PCR products sizing 314 bp are the control products (**Figure 27**).

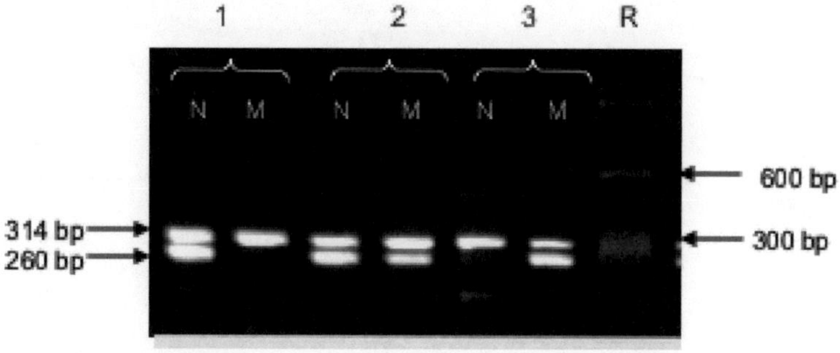

Figure 27.
ARMS-PCR for identifying β^E mutation. The 314-bp amplified products are internal control. The 260-bp amplified products are the β^E specific products. Sample #3 is homozygote for β^E mutation as the 260-pb amplified products are seen in only "M-reaction." Sample #1 is negative for the β^E mutation since the 260-bp amplified products are seen in only "N-reaction." Sample #2 is heterozygote for the β^E mutation since the 260-bp amplified products are seen in both "M-reaction" and "N-reaction."

Interpretation: Both M and N-reactions must have the 314-bp control products and the results can be read. If both M- and N-reactions have 260-bp PCR products, the samples are heterozygote for β^E with genotype of either β^E/β^A or β^E/β^T (A represents HbA; T represents other types of β-globin gene mutation). If the 260-bp PCR products are seen in only M-reaction, the samples are homozygote for β^E with genotype β^E/β^E. If samples have the 260-bp PCR products in only N-reaction, the samples are negative for the β^E with genotypes of either β^A/β^A or β^T/β^T (A represents HbA; T represents other types of β-globin gene mutation) (**Figure 27**).

9. Identification of β-thalassemia and HbE by MAS-PCR

This PCR technique was established by author and named multiplex allele specific (MAS)-PCR [29]. MAS was intended to be used for identifying $\beta^{Thalassemia}$ and β^E-mutations in samples that have already been diagnosed to be β-thalassemia carrier, HbE carrier, and SEA-α thalassemia 1 carrier. Therefore, only mutant primers are put together in this MAS-PCR. However, the internal control of this PCR protocol is the amplified products generated by the normal pair of primers for α-globin gene cluster.

Procedure: The PCR was performed in a total volume of 25 μL containing 1.1–1.4 ng genomic DNA, 140 μM dNTPs, 0.1 unit/μL of DNA polymerase, 0.25 ng/μL "Beta-common-multiplex" primer (5′-AAG AGC CAA GGA CAG GTA CGG CTG T-3′), 0.125 ng/μL "Beta-17-multiplex" primer (5′-CCA ACT TCA TCC ACG TTC ACG TA-3′), 0.125 ng/μL "Beta cds-41/42-multiplex" primer (5′-AGA TCC CCA AAG GAC TCA ACC T-3′), 0.125 ng/μL "Beta-E-multiplex" primer (5′-CGT ACC AAC CTG CCC AGG GCC AT-3′), 25 ng/μL "SEA-1-multiplex" primer (5′-TGA CTC CAA TAA ATG GAT GAG GA-3′), 0.25 ng/μL "SEA-2-multiplex" primer (5′-GCC TGC GCC GGG GAA CGT AAC CA-3′)and 0.5 ng/μL "SEA-3-multiplex" primer (5′-CGC CAA AGA TGG CTA CTC GGA GA-3′) in 10 mM Tris-HCl (pH 8.8), 50 mM KCl, 2.0% DMSO and 2.0 mM $MgCl_2$.

Thermal cycles: A total of 37 thermal cycles were carried out with each cycle comprising denaturation at 95°C for 1 min, primer annealing at 62°C for 30 s, and primer extension at 72°C for 30 s. Initial denaturation was extended to 5 min and final extension was prolonged to 7 min.

Detection of amplified products: The PCR products were separated via 2.0% agarose gel electrophoresis and visualized by the UV-transilluminator (**Figure 28**).

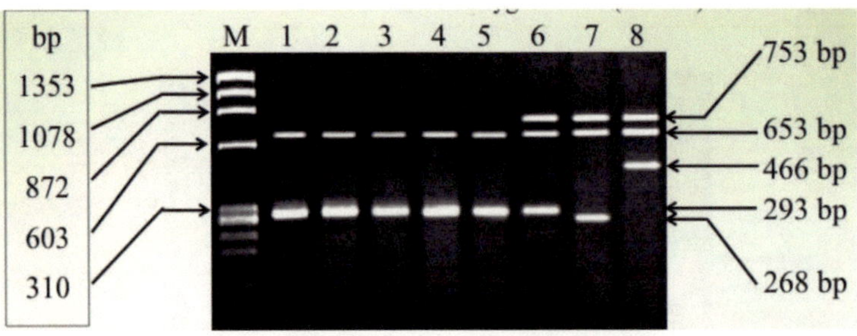

Figure 28.
MAS-PCR for identifying β-thalassemia mutation, β^E-mutation, and SEA-α thalassemia 1 mutation. The 653-bp amplified products are the internal control generated by the α-globin gene cluster specific oligonucleotide primers. Lanes 1–5 are positive for β^E mutation as the 293-bp amplified products are seen. Lane 6 is positive for both SEA-α thalassemia 1 and β^E mutations as both 753-bp amplified products and 293-bp amplified products are seen. Lane 7 is positive for both SEA-α thalassemia 1 and β^{17} mutation as both 753-bp amplified products and 268-bp amplified products are seen. Finally, lane 8 is positive for SEA-α thalassemia 1 and $\beta^{41/42}$ mutation as both 753-bp amplified products and 466-bp amplified products are seen (modified from [82]).

Interpretation: All reactions must have the 653-bp control products. Presence of 753-bp product indicates presence of the SEA-α thalassemia 1. Presence of the 466-bp, 293-bp, and 268-bp products indicates presence of $\beta^{41/42}$, β^{E}, and β^{17}, respectively (**Figure 28**).

10. Pitfalls in laboratory diagnosis of β-thalassemia and HbE

There are several pitfalls to be concerned when using laboratory data in diagnosis of β-thalassemia and HbE. The pitfalls are in both screening and confirmatory steps of laboratory diagnosis.

HbE tube test relies on concentration of NaCl. Therefore, exact amount of NaCl in the reagent must be prepared following the suggested ingredient. False positive results will be obtained if NaCl concentration is too high, and *vice versa.*

HbE screen test relies on pH-based microcolumn chromatography. Therefore, exact pH of buffer in the test kit must also be prepared. Too high pH causes falsely negative results and *vice versa.*

10.1 Pitfalls in screening tests for β-thalassemia and HbE carriers

1. **Pitfalls in one-tube osmotic fragility test (OFT).** The concentration of reagent must be exactly 0.36 and 0.45%, otherwise false positive results will be obtained if concentration is over 0.36 or over 0.45%. In contrast, false negative results will be obtained if concentration is less than 0.36 or 0.45%. Anemic blood samples will also give positive results. Therefore, Hb/Hct must also be checked if the results are positive. Not all HbE carriers have positive OFT results. Therefore, blood samples having negative OFT results must also be sent for HbE screen.

2. **Pitfalls in MCV and MCH evaluation.** MCV/MCH are the numeric data that must be obtained from automated blood cell counters that have good quality control. MCV must be obtained using fresh blood, but MCH may be obtained using 1 week-old blood. MCV is directly measured in automated blood counter, while MCH is generated by calculation. Thus, if blood samples have high degree of variation of red blood cell sizes or anisocytosis, false MCV values may be obtained. This situation may be found in β-thalassemia carriers or HbE carriers with co-existence iron deficiency anemia during treatment. Not all HbE carriers have MCV/MCH values below cutoff points. Therefore, all blood samples sent for MCV/MCH determination must also be sent for HbE screen. Most importantly, some blood samples may have discordant MCV-OFT results. It is then highly recommended to perform both OFT and MCV/MCH for screening for β-thalassemia and HbE carriers.

3. **Pitfalls in HbE screening test.** DCIP test is based on using the oxidizing reagent; dichlorophenolindophenol. This reagent can be reduced over long storage and the screening results will be falsely negative. Therefore, if color of the DCIP reagent turns deeply blue, it should not be used. HbH also denatured in the DCIP reagent. Therefore, positive samples must be checked if they are HbH disease.

10.2 Pitfalls in confirmatory tests for β-thalassemia and HbE

Normal hemoglobin type depends on age of the patients. Thus, reading and interpreting the hemoglobin typing results by all methodologies, age of the patients must be taken into account. In addition, transfused blood interferes the real hemoglobin typing results of the patients. If the patients of β-thalassemia disease (β^O/β^O) have just received blood transfusion, their hemoglobin types will be A_2AF, instead of A_2F which is the real hemoglobin type of the β^O/β^O. If patients of HbE/β^O-thalassemia (β^E/β^O) have recent blood transfusion, their hemoglobin types will be EFA, instead of EF which is the real hemoglobin type of β^O/β^E. Therefore, recent blood transfusion should always be taken into account when reading and interpreting the hemoglobin typing results.

Co-existence of α-thalassemia 1 in β-thalassemia carrier and in HbE carrier can be found some regions. This is called double α-thalassemia 1/β-thalassemia carriers and double α-thalassemia 1 and HbE carriers. Results of one-tube osmotic fragility test are always positive in double α-thalassemia 1/β-thalassemia carriers, being the same as that of the single β-thalassemia carrier. However, MCV/MCH in double α-thalassemia 1/β-thalassemia carriers are slightly higher than those in the single β-thalassemia carriers (70.7 ± 2.6 vs. 68.4 ± 2.7 for MCV, 21.0 ± 1.2 vs. 20.7 ± 0.9 for MCH) [83]. HbA_2 level in double α-thalassemia 1/β-thalassemia carriers is lower than that in single β-thalassemia carrier (5.27 ± 0.77% vs. 5.65 ± 0.78%) [29]. In contrast, the results of one-tube osmotic fragility test of double α-thalassemia 1/HbE carrier are usually positive, being different from those of single HbE which can be either positive or negative. The MCV/MCH in double α-thalassemia 1/HbE carrier are lower than those of the single HbE carrier (68.7 ± 8.9 fL vs. 75.7 ± 7.5 fL for MCV, 22.5 ± 3.1 pg vs. 24.9 ± 2.8 pg for MCH). HbE level in double α-thalassemia 1/HbE carrier are lower than those of the single HbE carrier (22.8 ± 4.4% vs. 27.6 ± 3.3%) [84]. Therefore, if HbE carriers have low HbE levels as well as MCV/MCH, further identification of α-thalassemia 1 genotype must be done.

11. Conclusions

Diagnosis of β-thalassemia and HbE requires laboratory investigations. Screening tests are used to search for carriers, while confirmatory tests are carried out in those samples positive for screening tests with the aim to make the definite diagnosis. There are several pitfalls in these laboratory tests, both in screening tests and confirmatory tests that must not be overlooked, otherwise misdiagnosis will occur.

Acknowledgements

The author thanks Mr. Eaktong Limveeraprachak of Sawan Pracharak Hospital, Nakorn Sawan Province, Thailand for providing hemoglobin typing results put in this chapter.

Conflict of interest

The authors declare no conflict of interest.

Author details

Thanusak Tatu
Division of Clinical Microscopy, Department of Medical Technology, Faculty of Associated Medical Sciences, Chiang Mai University, Chiang Mai, Thailand

*Address all correspondence to: tthanu@hotmail.com; thanusak.t@cmu.ac.th

References

[1] Weatherall DJ, Clegg JB. The Thalassaemia Syndromes. 4th ed. Oxford: Blackwell Scientific; 2001

[2] Flint J, Harding RM, Boyce AJ, Clegg JB. The population genetics of the haemoglobinopathies. In: Rodgers GP, editor. Bailliere's Clinical Haematology, International Practice and Research: Sickle Cell Disease and Thalassaemia. Vol. 11. London: Bailliere Tindall; 1998. pp. 1-51

[3] Higgs DR, Weatherall DJ. The alpha thalassaemias. Cellular and Molecular Life Sciences. 2009;**66**(7):1154-1162

[4] Olivieri NF. The beta-thalassemias. The New England Journal of Medicine. 1999;**341**(2):99-109

[5] Fucharoen S, Winichagoon P. Hemoglobinopathies in Southeast Asia: Molecular biology and clinical medicine. Hemoglobin. 1997;**21**(4):299-319

[6] Thein SL. Genetic modifiers of beta-thalassemia. Haematologica. 2005;**90**(5):649-660

[7] Laosombat V, Wongchanchailert M, Sattayasevana B, Wiriyasateinkul A, Fucharoen S. Clinical and hematological features of beta(+)-thalassemia (IVS-1 nt 5, G-C mutation) in Thai patients. European Journal of Haematology. 2001;**67**(2):100-104

[8] Laosombat V, Wongchanchailert M, Sattayasevana B, Wiriyasateinkul A, Fucharoen S. Clinical and hematological features of codon 17, A-T mutation of beta-thalassemia in Thai patients. European Journal of Haematology. 2001;**66**(2):126-129

[9] Laosombat V, Wongchanchailert M, Sattayasevana B, Wiriyasateinkul A, Fucharoen S. Clinical and hematologic features of beta0-thalassemia (frameshift 41/42 mutation) in Thai patients. Haematologica. 2001;**86**(2):138-141

[10] Weatherall DJ. Hemoglobin E beta-thalassemia: An increasingly common disease with some diagnostic pitfalls. The Journal of Pediatrics. 1998;**132**(5):765-767

[11] Fucharoen S, Weatherall DJ. The hemoglobin E thalassemias. Cold Spring Harbor Perspectives in Medicine. 2012;**2**(8):1-15

[12] Rees DC, Styles L, Vichinsky EP, Clegg JB, Weatherall DJ. The hemoglobin E syndromes. Annals of the New York Academy of Sciences. 1998;**850**:334-343

[13] Winichagoon P, Thitivichianlert A, Lebnak T, Piankijagum A, Fucharoen S. Screening for the carriers of thalassemias and abnormal hemoglobins at the community level. The Southeast Asian Journal of Tropical Medicine and Public Health. 2002;**33**(Suppl 2):145-150

[14] Wiwanitkit V, Suwansaksri J, Paritpokee N. Combined one-tube osmotic fragility (OF) test and dichlorophenol-indolphenol (DCIP) test screening for hemoglobin disorders, an experience in 213 Thai pregnant women. Clinical Laboratory. 2002;**48**(9-10):525-528

[15] Tatu T, Kasinrerk W. A novel test tube method of screening for hemoglobin E. International Journal of Laboratory Hematology. 2012;**34**(1):59-64

[16] Wanapirak C, Sirichotiyakul S, Luewan S, Srisupundit K, Tongsong T. Comparison of the accuracy of dichlorophenolindophenol (DCIP), modified DCIP, and hemoglobin E tests to screen for the HbE trait in pregnant women. International Journal of Gynaecology and Obstetrics. 2009;**107**(1):59-60

[17] Papassotiriou I, Traeger-Synodios J, Vlachou C, Karagiorga M, Metaxotou A, Kanavakis E, et al. Rapid and accurate quantitation of Hb Bart's and Hb H using weak cation exchange high performance liquid chromatography: Correlation with the α-thalassemia genotype. Hemoglobin. 1999;**23**(3):203-211

[18] Sanguansermsri T, Thanarattanakorn P, Steger HF, Tongsong T, Chanprapaph P, Wanpirak C, et al. Prenatal diagnosis of beta-thalassemia major by high-performance liquid chromatography analysis of hemoglobins in fetal blood samples. Hemoglobin. 2001;**25**(1):19-27

[19] Fucharoen S, Winichagoon P, Wisedpanichkij R, Sae-Ngow B, Sriphanich R, Oncoung W, et al. Prenatal and postnatal diagnoses of thalassemias and hemoglobinopathies by HPLC. Clinical Chemistry. 1998;**44**(4):740-748

[20] Chambers K, Phillips A, Chapman CS. Use of a low pressure liquid chromatography system for haemoglobinopathy screening. Clinical and Laboratory Haematology. 1993;**15**(2):119-128

[21] Kuesap J, Chaijaroenkul W, Rungsihirunrat K, Pongjantharasatien K, Na-Bangchang K. Coexistence of malaria and thalassemia in malaria endemic areas of Thailand. The Korean Journal of Parasitology. 2015;**53**(3):265-270

[22] Pornprasert S, Kongthai K, Waneesorn J, Jaiping K, Treesuwan K. Development of control material for hemoglobin analysis. Clinical Chemistry and Laboratory Medicine. 2011;**50**(2): 351-356

[23] Jenkins M, Ratnaike S. Capillary electrophoresis of hemoglobin. Clinical Chemistry and Laboratory Medicine. 2003;**41**(6):747-754

[24] Jenkins MA, Hendy J, Smith IL. Evaluation of hemoglobin A2 quantitation assay and hemoglobin variant screening by capillary electrophoresis. Journal of Capillary Electrophoresis. 1997;**4**(3):137-143

[25] Sangkitporn S, Sangkitporn SK, Tanjatham S, Suwannakan B, Rithapirom S, Yodtup C, et al. Multicenter validation of fully automated capillary electrophoresis method for diagnosis of thalassemias and hemoglobinopathies in Thailand. The Southeast Asian Journal of Tropical Medicine and Public Health. 2011;**42**(5):1224-1232

[26] Shihabi ZK, Hinsdale ME, Daugherty HK Jr. Hemoglobin A2 quantification by capillary zone electrophoresis. Electrophoresis. 2000;**21**(4):749-752

[27] Winichagoon P, Svasti S, Munkongdee T, Chaiya W, Boonmongkol P, Chantrakul N, et al. Rapid diagnosis of thalassemias and other hemoglobinopathies by capillary electrophoresis system. Translational Research. 2008;**152**(4):178-184

[28] Kerdpoo S, Laopajon W, Kasinrerk W, Pata S, Tatu T. A modified sandwich ELISA for accurate measurement of HbF in alpha-thalassemia carriers containing Hb Bart's and Hb Portland 1. Journal of Immunoassay & Immunochemistry. 2018;**39**(3):323-336

[29] Tatu T, Kiewkarnkha T, Khuntarak S, Khamrin S, Suwannasin S, Kasinrerk W. Screening for co-existence of alpha-thalassemia in beta-thalassemia and in HbE heterozygotes via an enzyme-linked immunosorbent assay for Hb Bart's and embryonic zeta-globin chain. International Journal of Hematology. 2012;**95**(4):386-393

[30] Kuntaruk S, Tatu T, Keowkarnkah T, Kasinrerk W. Sandwich ELISA for hemoglobin A2 quantification and identification of beta-thalassemia

carriers. International Journal of Hematology. 2010;**91**(2):219-228

[31] Thorpe SJ, Thein SL, Sampietro M, Craig JE, Mahon B, Huehns ER. Immunochemical estimation of haemoglobin types in red blood cells by FACS analysis. British Journal of Haematology. 1994;**87**(1):125-132

[32] Tayapiwatana C, Kuntaruk S, Tatu T, Chiampanichayakul S, Munkongdee T, Winichagoon P, et al. Simple method for screening of alpha-thalassaemia 1 carriers. International Journal of Hematology. 2009;**89**(5):559-567

[33] Old JM, Varawalla NY, Weatherall DJ. Rapid detection and prenatal diagnosis of beta-thalassaemia: Studies in Indian and Cypriot populations in the UK. Lancet. 1990;**336**(8719):834-837

[34] Chang JG, Lu JM, Huang JM, Chen JT, Liu HJ, Chang CP. Rapid diagnosis of beta-thalassaemia by mutagenically separated polymerase chain reaction (MS-PCR) and its application to prenatal diagnosis. British Journal of Haematology. 1995;**91**(3):602-607

[35] Rust S, Funke H, Assmann G. Mutagenically separated PCR (MS-PCR): A highly specific one step procedure for easy mutation detection. Nucleic Acids Research. 1993;**21**(16):3623-3629

[36] Sritong W, Tatu T, Saetung R, Sa-nguansermsri T. Rapid identification of β-thalassemia mutations by mutagenically separated polymerase chain reaction (MS-PCR). Chiangmai Medical Bulletin. 2004;**43**(4):133-141 (in Thai)

[37] He X, Sheng M, Xu M, Xiong C, Ren Z. Rapid identification of common β-thalassemia mutations in the Chinese population using duplex or triplex amplicon genotyping by high-resolution melting analysis. Genetic Testing and Molecular Biomarkers. 2010;**14**(6):851-856

[38] Lin M, Jiao JW, Zhan XH, Zhan XF, Pan MC, Wang JL, et al. High resolution melting analysis: A rapid screening and typing tool for common beta-thalassemia mutation in Chinese population. PLoS One. 2014;**9**(8):e102243

[39] Saetung R, Ongchai S, Charoenkwan P, Sanguansermsri T. Genotyping of beta thalassemia trait by high-resolution DNA melting analysis. The Southeast Asian Journal of Tropical Medicine and Public Health. 2013;**44**(6):1055-1064

[40] Kulapong P, Sanguansermsri T, Tawarat S, Mertz G. Dichlorophe-nolindophenol (DCIP) precipitation test. Bulletin of the Medical Technology Association. 1976;**9**(3):161

[41] Tatu T, Prakunwisit D, Chayajak S, Chiampanichayakul S, Kasinrerk W. RBC count and its differentiation potential between α-thalassemia (SEA type), β-thalassemia and HbE heterozygotes. Chiang Mai University (CMU) Journal of Natural Sciences. 2007;**6**(1):57-64

[42] Rund D, Filon D, Strauss N, Rachmilewitz EA, Oppenheim A. Mean corpuscular volume of heterozygotes for beta-thalassemia correlates with the severity of mutations. Blood. 1992;**79**(1):238-243

[43] Sirichotiyakul S, Maneerat J, Sa-nguansermsri T, Dhananjayanonda P, Tongsong T. Sensitivity and specificity of mean corpuscular volume testing for screening for alpha-thalassemia-1 and beta-thalassemia traits. The Journal of Obstetrics and Gynaecology Research. 2005;**31**(3):198-201

[44] Karimi M, Rasekhi AR. Efficiency of premarital screening of beta-thalassemia trait using MCH rather

than MCV in the population of Fars Province, Iran. Haematologia. 2002;**32**(2):129-133

[45] Yeo GS, Tan KH, Liu TC. Screening for beta thalassaemia and HbE traits with the mean red cell volume in pregnant women. Annals of the Academy of Medicine, Singapore. 1994;**23**(3):363-366

[46] Ittarat W, Ongcharoenjai S, Rayatong O, Pirat N. Correlation between some discrimination functions and hemoglobin E. Journal of the Medical Association of Thailand. 2000;**83**(3):259-265

[47] Chow J, Phelan L, Bain BJ. Evaluation of single-tube osmotic fragility as a screening test for thalassemia. American Journal of Hematology. 2005;**79**(3):198-201

[48] Bobhate SK, Gaikwad ST, Bhaledrao T. NESTROFT as a screening test for detection of β-thalassemia trait. Indian Journal of Pathology & Microbiology. 2002;**45**(3):265-267

[49] Mamtani M, Jawahirani A, Das K, Rughwani V, Kulkarni H. Bias-corrected diagnostic performance of the naked-eye single-tube red-cell osmotic fragility test (NESTROFT): An effective screening tool for beta-thalassemia. Hematology. 2006;**11**(4):277-286

[50] Fucharoen G, Sanchaisuriya K, Sae-ung N, Dangwibul S, Fucharoen S. A simplified screening strategy for thalassaemia and haemoglobin E in rural communities in South-East Asia. Bulletin of the World Health Organization. 2004;**82**(5):364-372

[51] Sanguansermsri T, Phumyu N, Chomchuen S, Steger HF. Screening for alpha-thalassemia-1 heterozygotes in expecting couples by the combination of a simple erythrocyte osmotic fragility test and a PCR-based method. Community Genetics. 1999;**2**(1):26-29

[52] Sanguansermsri T. Methods for Treatment and Prevention of Severe Thalassemia in Children. Wattachai: Chiang Mai; 1994 (in Thai)

[53] Tatu T. Techniques and Interpretation of Laboratory Tests for Thalassemia and Hemoglobinopathies. Darawan Printing: Chiang Mai; 2009 (in Thai)

[54] Tatu T, Sweatman D. Hemolysis area: A new parameter of erythrocyte osmotic fragility for screening of thalassemia trait. Journal of Laboratory Physicians. 2018;**10**(2):214-220

[55] Chapple L, Harris A, Phelan L, Bain BJ. Reassessment of a simple chemical method using DCIP for screening for haemoglobin E. Journal of Clinical Pathology. 2006;**59**(1):74-76

[56] Pilai S. Development of CMU-DCIP-FADE for Use in HbE Screen in Population. Chiang Mai: Chiang Mai University; 2004

[57] Sanguansermsri T, Sangkapreecha C, Steger HF. HbE screening test. Thai Journal of Hematology and Transfusion Medicine. 1998;**8**(3):215-221 (in Thai)

[58] Sirichotiyakul S, Tongprasert F, Tongsong T. Screening for hemoglobin E trait in pregnant women. International Journal of Gynaecology and Obstetrics. 2004;**86**(3):390-391

[59] The Working Party of the General Haematology Task Force of the British Committee for Standards in Haematology. The laboratory diagnosis of haemoglobinopathies. British Journal of Haematology. 1998;**101**(4):783-792

[60] Mosca A, Paleari R, Scime-Degani V, Leone L, Leone D, Ivaldi G. Inter-method differences and commutability of control materials for HbA2 measurement. Clinical Chemistry and Laboratory Medicine. 2000;**38**(10):997-1002

[61] Khadsongkram B. Developmemt of Naked Eye Microcolumn for HbE Screen (NEMES) for Screening of HbE Carriers. Chiang Mai: Chiang Mai University; 2008 (in Thai)

[62] Bunn HF, Forget BG, Ranney HM. Human Hemoglobins. Toronto: W.B. Saunders Company; 1977

[63] Mohammad AA, Okorodudu AO, Bissell MG, Dow P, Reger G, Meier A, et al. Clinical application of capillary isoelectric focusing on fused silica capillary for determination of hemoglobin variants. Clinical Chemistry. 1997;**43**(9):1798-1799

[64] Wood WG, Analysis H. In: Weatherall DJ, editor. The Thalassemia: Methods in Hematology. Vol. 6. New York: Churchill Livingstone; 1983. pp. 31-53

[65] Sitti W. Development of *In-house* Micro-Column Chromatography for Measuring HbA_2/E Levels Used to Detect β-Thalassemia Carrier and HbE Carrier. Chiang Mai: Chiang Mai University; 2007 (in Thai)

[66] Betke K, Marti HR, Schlicht I. Estimation of small percentages of foetal haemoglobin. Nature. 1959;**184**: 1877-1878

[67] Gupta PK, Kumar H, Kumar S, Jaiprakash M. Cation exchange high performance liquid chromatography for diagnosis of haemoglobinopathies. Medical Journal, Armed Forces India. 2009;**65**(1):33-37

[68] Tatu T, Gategasem P, Hathirat P. Hemoglobin typing by high performance liquid chromatography. The Southeast Asian Journal of Tropical Medicine and Public Health. 1997;**28**(2):417-423

[69] Viprakasit V, Ekwattanakit S. Clinical classification, screening and diagnosis for thalassemia. Hematology/Oncology Clinics of North America. 2018;**32**(2):193-211

[70] Tatu T, Wongchompoo P, Sakdasirisathaporn P, Nawarawong W. HbF and HbE levels in HbE/beta-o-thalassemia are heterogenous. Bulletin of Chiangmai Associated Medical Sciences Medical Science. 2011;**44**:17-23 (in Thai)

[71] Wang J, Zhou S, Huang W, Liu Y, Cheng C, Lu X, et al. CE-based analysis of hemoglobin and its applications in clinical analysis. Electrophoresis. 2006;**27**(15):3108-3124

[72] Gan YY, Lai CM, Lee SH, Gan LH. Production of monoclonal and polyclonal antibodies against various haemoglobins for the detection of thalassaemias. Annals of the Academy of Medicine, Singapore. 1996;**25**(1):75-78

[73] Jintaridth P, Srisomsap C, Vichittumaros K, Kalpravidh RW, Winichagoon P, Fucharoen S, et al. Chicken egg yolk antibodies specific for the gamma chain of human hemoglobin for diagnosis of thalassemia. International Journal of Hematology. 2006;**83**(5):408-414

[74] Shyamala M, Kiefer CR, Moscoso H, Garver FA. A monoclonal antibody-linked immunoassay for hemoglobin H disease. Annals of Hematology. 1992;**65**(1):37-40

[75] Winichagoon P, Kumpan P, Holmes P, Finlayson J, Newbound C, Kabral A, et al. Validation of the immunochromatographic strip for alpha-thalassemia screening: A multicenter study. Translational Research. 2015;**165**(6):689-695

[76] Shyamala M, Kiefer CR, Moscoso H, Garver FA. Application of a monoclonal antibody specific for the delta chain of hemoglobin A_2 in the diagnosis of β thalassemia. American Journal of Hematology. 1991;**38**(3):214-219

[77] Needs T, Lynch DT. Beta Thalassemia. Treasure Island, FL: StatPearls; 2019

[78] Thein SL. Genetic basis and genetic modifiers of beta-thalassemia and sickle cell disease. Advances in Experimental Medicine and Biology. 2017;**1013**:27-57

[79] Old J, Varawalla NY, Weatherall DJ. Rapid detection and prenatal diagnosis of β-thalassemia: Studies in Indian and Cypriot population in the UK. Lancet. 1990;**336**:834-837

[80] Sritong W, Tatu T, Saetung R, Sanguansermsri T. Rapid identification of β-thalassemia mutations by mutagenically separated polymerase chain reaction. Chiangmai Medical Bulletin. 2004;**43**(4):133-141

[81] Sirichotiyakul S, Saetung R, Sanguansermsri T. Analysis of β-thalassemia mutations in northern Thailand using an automated fluorescence DNA sequencing technique. Hemoglobin. 2003;**27**(2):89-95

[82] Suwannasin S. Study of Molecular Background of Hematologically Silent α-Thalassemia and Development of Polymerase Chain Reaction to Detect Double Heterozygous α/β Thalassemia Commonly Found in Thais. Chiang Mai University: Chiang Mai University; 2009

[83] Tatu T, Sayachak S, Chiampanichayakul S, Kasinrerk W, Piyamongkol W. Red blood cell parameters and Hb Bart's levels in simple β-and double α/β-thalassemia heterozygotes. In: Thai Society of Hematology Annual Meeting March 26-29, 2006; The Royal Golden Jubilee Building, Bangkok. 2006

[84] Leckngam P, Limweeraprajak E, Kiewkarnkha T, Tatu T. The Hb E (HBB: c.79G>A), mean corpuscular volume, mean corpuscular hemoglobin cutoff points in double heterozygous Hb E/− −(SEA) alpha-Thalassemia-1 carriers are dependent on hemoglobin levels. Hemoglobin. 2017;**41**(1):38-43